ANXIETY

A Self Help Guide to Control Depression, Manage Stress, Overcome Anger, Calm Your Anxious Mind, Improve Self-esteem and Boost Self Confidence

(Hack and Rewire Your Brain)

Scott M. Pittman

D1555598

Published by Kevin Dennis

Anxiety Relief: A Self Help Guide to Control Depression, Manage Stress, Overcome Anger, Calm Your Anxious Mind, Improve Self-esteem and Boost Self Confidence (Hack and Rewire Your Brain)

ISBN 978-1-989920-79-4

Legal & Disclaimer

The information contained in this book is not designed to replace or take the place of any form of medicine or professional medical advice. The information in this book has been provided for educational and entertainment purposes only.

The information contained in this book has been compiled from sources deemed reliable, and it is accurate to the best of the Author's knowledge; however, the Author cannot guarantee its accuracy and validity and cannot be held liable for any errors or omissions. Changes are periodically made to this book. You must consult your doctor or get professional medical advice before using any of the suggested remedies, techniques, or information in this book.

TABLE OF CONTENTS

INTRODUCTION..1

CHAPTER 1: DISCOVER YOUR PERSONALITY 3

CHAPTER 2: THE CAUSE OF ANXIETY................................ 13

BIOLOGICAL EXPLANATION 13

CHAPTER 3: COMMON TRIGGERS & HOW TO AVOID THEM
.... 23

CHAPTER 4: TYPES OF MEDITATION 28

CHAPTER 5: DEALING WITH SEPARATION ANXIETY 34

CHAPTER 6: IDENTIFYING THE PHYSICAL, EMOTIONAL AND
BEHAVIORAL MANIFESTATIONS OF ANXIETY 40

CHAPTER 7: RECOGNIZING SOCIAL ANXIETY AND SOCIAL
PHOBIA 43

CHAPTER 8: MANAGING STRESS....................................... 51

CHAPTER 9: SOCIALLY SCARED IS COMMON.................... 56

CHAPTER 10: WHAT TYPE ARE YOU? 69

CHAPTER 11: DETOX, HOW TO REMOVE THE PHYSICAL
CAUSES OF ANXIETY... 71

CHAPTER 12: EVIDENCE-BASED ANALYSIS 77

CHAPTER 13: BIPOLAR DISORDER TREATMENT OPTIONS 80

CHAPTER 14: GENERALIZED ANXIETY DISORDER: WHEN WORRY GETS OUT OF CONTROL...................................... 86

CHAPTER 15: SIGNS AND SYMPTOMS............................. 93

CHAPTER 16: TREATING SOCIAL ANXIETY 97

CHAPTER 17: WHAT IS ANXIETY DISORDER?................. 101

CHAPTER 18: SYMPTOMS OF ANXIETY DISORDER AND PANIC ATTACKS... 110

CHAPTER 19: SELF-HELP FOR CURING ANXIETY DISORDERS 116

CHAPTER 20: PERSISTENCE, DISCIPLINE AND POTENTIAL 127

CHAPTER 21: DIET AND EXERCISE 129

CHAPTER 22: A BRIEF LOOK AT MEDITATIVE PRACTICES 133

CHAPTER 23: UNDERSTANDING THE SYMPTOMS AND CAUSES OF ANXIETY 139

CHAPTER 24: HOW TO PERFORM BASIC TAPPING 149

CHAPTER 25: HOW TO APPLY AROMATHERAPY TO YOUR EVERYDAY LIFE 157

CHAPTER 26: LEARNING TO FOLLOW THROUGH............ 167

CHAPTER 27: SYMPTOMS OF AND CAUSES OF ANXIETY DISORDERS.. 170

CHAPTER 28: NUTRITIONAL METHODS OF DEALING WITH ANXIETY 173

CHAPTER 29: WAYS TO REDUCE STRESS AND ANXIETY.. 177

CONCLUSION.. 181

Introduction

This book contains proven steps and strategies on how to minimize anxiety so you can put yourself at peace. Anxiety is the unpleasant state of inner turmoil, most often accompanied by nervous behaviour such as rumination, somatic complaints, and pacing back and forth. Anxiety is not the same as fear; it is rather the subjectively unpleasant feelings of dread over anticipated events, like the feeling of imminent death.

Every moment the working day concludes, there is a chance you could experience anxiety. Whether or not you suffer anxiety disorder, you can't allow anxiety to rule and control over your life and the happiness you deserve. The reality is: anxiety, no matter how bad, can affect your life in negative ways. Why would you rob yourself of great happiness and amazing productivity? I certainly wouldn't.

There is a mass of info and many new treatments we come across daily to help cope with anxiety and heaps of them stay very tempting to compel anyone to abandon what is being doing towards pursuing them instead. While I cannot promise that this book will resolve all your anxiety problems, I can promise it would tackle the matters necessary to help you move forward and set the foundation for an anxiety-free life.

Thanks again for downloading this book, I hope you enjoy it!

Chapter 1: Discover Your Personality

It's time to stop and wonder... Why do some people like putting on make-up, or working out at the gym, or going to parties, while others like sitting on the couch and reading a book? Why do some people love to share embarrassing moments, while others... really get embarrassed about it? Why is it that some people can't say no to a challenge, love extreme sports, and will follow someone out into the parking lot to continue a debate, while others couldn't care less?

On a different note... Is self-improvement possible? If someone is bothered by their weaknesses, is there any GOOD plan out there to help? Why is it so hard to change? What is it people need to change? Understanding a little about personality answers all of these questions. Discovering your personality is the key to real self-improvement. It lets you understand better why you are the way you are... why you think the way you think and act the way you act. This empowers you to change, to improve yourself.

Once you know they way you work, you also discover how to make yourself work the way you want to work. Take cooking as an example. If you want to change a recipe, you need to first know the ingredients. People are the same way. If you want to change yourself, you first need to know the elements that affect how you act. Then, you can decide what is good, and what you want to add or take out to become better. Learning about personality can also help you understand how others think, and why some of them think differently from you. In addition to helping with self-knowledge and improvement, understanding personality, will also improve your relationships with others.

What is PERSONALITY?

There are numerous meanings to the word personality, but the one that applies to personality as used in this e Book, is: "the complex or characteristics that distinguishes an individual or nation or group, especially the totality of an individual's behavioral and emotional characteristics; a set of distinctive traits and characteristics".

Elements of Personality

There are four main personality types, or groups: choleric, sanguine, melancholic, and phlegmatic. Everyone falls into one of these main groups, or a combination of two of them. Remember: each persona is individual and unique, with special strengths and weaknesses. No personality type is better than any other. Within each personality type, there are many variations, and no two people, even people with the same personality type, are the same. There are as many personality variations as there are people. The personality groups are a guide, a way to know and understand yourself and others better.

Three main elements define the personality types:

Introverted/Extroverted

An introverted person lives within their own minds. They think they reflect and ponder. They tend to be more private people, more quiet people. They like the comfort of their home, and close group of friends. They like having alone time once in a while, so they have time to just think and sort through their thought and emotions.

An extroverted person, on the other hand, lives to be with people. They love to go out, to talk, to be at parties, to hear what other people have to say. While an introverted person thinks things through, and extroverted person talks them through. If an extroverted person is asked a question, that they've never thought of before, they may say, "I don't know," and then proceed to talk aloud nonstop until they reach their conclusion, or are distracted about something else. The extroverted person finds their fulfillment in being with people, and have a hard time being alone. Even when working on their own, they would rather work in a room with other people than by themselves.

People centered/principle centered

This element refers to what influences each person in making large decisions.

Some people are principle centered. They have different ideas, values, and principles that govern all of their decisions. If something is coherent with their principles, it is worth doing and supporting. If it conflicts with their principles, it is something to be fought against, or simply not supported. People who are principle centered will act based on their principles regardless of what other people think, and sometimes, regardless of how other people are affected.

People centered people are the opposite. They base the decisions and actions very much based on what other people think. For them, the first value is pleasing the person. People centered personalities often don't have their principles thought out or expressed as thoroughly as principle centered personalities. Even when their principles are called into question, people persons are more likely to bend principle in order to please people. Principle centered personalities bend people to please principle. As we will see later, when discussing the different character types, both forms of influence have positive and negative points.

Primary/Secondary

A primary person acts first and thinks later - sometimes to their dismay. The primary person is quick to reach conclusions, quick to act, quick to feel, and quick to forget and move on. Their emotional resonance is sharp and intense, but frequently short lived. The primary person can go from laughing to crying to angry, and back to laughing again in a short period of time.

A secondary person thinks firsts, and acts later. They take longer to reflect, decide, act, and respond... but their response, particularly their mental and emotional response is of a longer, steadier duration.

Personality Types:

The four personality types combine these elements in the following way:

Choleric: extroverted, principle centered, primary

Sanguine: extroverted, people centered, primary

Melancholic: introverted, people centered, secondary

Phlegmatic: introverted, principle centered, secondary

PERSONALITY TYPES AND HOW TO MOTIVATE THEM TO GET THEIR BEST SUPPORTS

Did you know that some horses will follow you for a carrot, while other horses won't budge unless you whack them with a stick? Well, people are also motivated by either carrots, or sticks. Some people move towards goals. Other people move away from consequences.

As earlier mentioned, psychologists have identified four distinct personality types: Sanguine, Phlegmatic, Melancholic and Choleric. Everyone leans towards one of these types. If you learn to understand what excites, motivates, irritates and frustrates these different personality types, you'll be well on your way to understanding why certain people frustrate you more than others.

Sanguine and Choleric personalities tend to be fast-paced and impulsive. If you dangle a carrot in front of them, they'll probably jump at the carrot. On the other hand, Phlegmatic and Melancholic personalities tend to be slower-paced and indecisive. To get them into gear, you sometimes have to show them the sticky consequences of not taking a risk.

"Carrot" people go to the dentist because they want white teeth. "Stick" people go to the dentist because they don't want cavities. "Carrot" people try new things because they want to get ahead and be in the know. "Stick" people try new things because they don't want to fall behind, or mess things up.

Can you see the difference?

Here's another personality trait that you should consider. Melancholic and Choleric personalities tend to be internally validated. In other words, they carry inside themselves a strong sense of their own opinions and their own sense of right. If you give Cholerics too much feedback, they'll ask you to mind your own business. If you give Melancholics illogical feedback, they'll throw their hands up in frustration.

In contrast, Sanguine and Phlegmatic personalities tend to be externally validated. Meaning, they need people to validate them, and they only thrive when others support them. In fact, they often value your opinion more than they value their own. If you don't give a Sanguine enough feedback, you'll likely be tracked down and asked what you think; while Phlegmatics can't make a decision without considering how everyone around them is affected by the decision.

Basically, Melancholic and Choleric personalities tend to make decisions based upon what they think, want, or need; while Phlegmatic and Sanguine personalities tend to make decisions based upon what others think, want, or need. That being the case, whenever you want to present a solution, opinion, or idea to someone, you should probably consider that person's personality type because unless your solution motivates his or her type, you're wasting your time and confusing the issue.

Whatever personality type you're dealing with, you make your most effective and persuasive presentations when you show each type how they can get what they want by agreeing to work with you...

Chapter 2: The Cause Of Anxiety

Biological Explanation

The nature versus nurture debate is often a hot topic among researchers and clinicians. Many types of research support the view that genes have an influence on anxiety in individuals. Anxiety disorders often run in families. There is some evidence that, along with genes, early childhood environment or learning experiences within families seem to make some people more vulnerable to anxiety disorders than others.

The search for specific genes related to anxiety disorders is in the preliminary phase. Consider this: Researchers analyzed the genetic make-up of 1,065 families of which some individuals had OCD, and found that the gene in question was not associated with the disease. However, in the May 2014 issue of the journal, *Molecular Psychiatry*, their paper drew upon other research to conclude that there still may be a link between individuals' DNA code and the occurrence of OCD, but these ideas still required further investigation.

For most people, genetic risk for anxiety is less likely to be an automatic 'on' switch than a complicated mix of genes that can put you at risk for *developing* anxiety. Even with a genetic predisposition, your anxiety disorder might be different from your relatives' anxiety in important ways.

A genetic predisposition to anxiety could start young. Studies have shown that when anxiety develops in an individual before age 20, close relatives are more likely to have anxiety as well. A study published in the June 2013 issue of the *Journal of Anxiety Disorders* underscored that certain anxiety traits correlated with panic disorder became evident in a child by age 8.

Researchers have tried to better understand the genetics behind anxiety disorders by examining whether relatives have the same anxiety disorder. They have found that people whose twins have it are at a *significantly greater* risk for panic disorder and people whose first-degree relatives have it, such as a parent or sibling, are at a *somewhat greater* risk for panic disorder.

Studies showed that the risk of anxiety tends to run in families, but the role of genetic influence versus the influence of the family environment remains unclear, concluded researchers in an article published in the June 2011 issue of the *Journal of Korean Medical Science*. As it stands now, experts believe the genes involved may modify your emotional responses in a way that might lead to anxiety. Whether two people with a similar mix of genes develop anxiety or not could depend on their experiences or environmental risk factors.

Environmental Explanation

Anxiety is one of the most common mental health issues across the world but Gen Z has been especially vulnerable to it. Teenagers, kids, and young adults from the newest generation are faced with dire prospects in terms of economy, inequality, and other issues. As teens become more aware of these problems, they also seem to develop higher levels of anxiety. Up to 80% of the younger generation have significant degrees of worry and anxiety in regards to their future, jobs, and terrorism, and the numbers seem to be growing (Hertz, 2016).

However, while the world around us has its issues, a significant factor contributing to the anxiety of the new generation may be the anxiety of their parents. Even when factors, such as financial difficulties serve as important contributors to the anxiety of the younger generations, parents remain one of the biggest influences on their development and emotional state. Studies have determined that parents often model anxious behaviors and thoughts for their children, so when parents act anxiously, children are more likely to do the same (Burstein & Ginsburg, 2010). Parents with anxiety disorders tended to act in specific ways since their children were young and might, inadvertently, expose the child to higher levels of criticism or doubt, which can also influence them negatively (Budinger, Drazdowski & Ginsburg, 2013) and contribute to a higher level of anxiety as they grow older.

What does this mean? Parents who hope that their children will not have to live with anxiety might want to evaluate their own anxiety levels, behaviors, and thoughts that might be transferred to the next generation and work to reduce their own anxiety first.

Another explanation for increased anxiety may be smartphone and internet use. Excessive smartphone use could cause increased anxiety and isolation in teenagers. Teens interact with peers via smartphone more often than they do in person.

To add to this factor, teenage girls have been observed to tend to judge themselves based on what social media displays. Some researchers speculate that girls and women are continually bombarded by media messages, dominant culture, and humor. Girls have constant online connections via texting, Instagram, and Snapchat. They are subject to the harsh focus on looks and other judgments these social media platforms can exacerbate. Boys tend to play computer and video games more often than interacting with social media. This may explain why girls may be more vulnerable to anxiety.

Many girls may develop their "entire identity" from their phone, constantly checking Instagram photos, Snapchat stories and the number of tags and likes received.

Life Transitions and Developmental Issues

Changes in life, whether expected or unexpected, can be significantly disorienting. Though we all experience change on a consistent basis, the process of a big transition can be particularly overwhelming. Some girls may develop anxiety disorders due to specific stressors that are tied to life transitions and developmental stages.

Each developmental stage presents particular tasks. In childhood, a girl's developmental tasks involve socialization, family relationships, friendships, and school performance. A crisis may arise from peer conflict, loss of friends through relocation, conflict with parents, school difficulties, and entering school during early childhood.

During the teen years from age 13 to 18, the hormones kick in, peer pressures escalate and academic expectations increase. Throughout adolescence, a person's tasks center on identity issues. A crisis may arise from performance in academics or athletics, graduation from high school, entering college, conflicts with parents over personal habits and lifestyle, break-ups with boyfriends or girlfriends, sexual orientation conflict, an unwanted pregnancy, career indecision, and challenges at a first job.

Girls with anxiety disorders may exhibit low energy and concentration difficulties which, in turn, lead to poor attendance, a drop in grades, and frustration with schoolwork. Anxiety can take a huge emotional toll, and depression often sets in. They may experience irritability, anger, and agitation. Other symptoms may include unexplained aches and pains, extreme sensitivity to criticism, withdrawal from certain people, lethargy, and continuous, unrelenting unhappiness. There are no conclusive explanations as to why anxiety and depression so often coexist, according to the Anxiety and Depression Association of America. Anxiety affects women and men differently. The fight or flight response in the female brain system is activated more readily and remains longer than in men due to the presence of estrogen and progesterone.

Among young adults from age 18 to 34, women's concerns center on intimacy, starting a career or occupation, and parenthood. Potential crisis events include rejection by a partner, unwanted pregnancy, birth of a child, inability to have children, extramarital affair, separation or divorce, illness in a child, discipline problems with children, inability to manage demands of parenthood, academic difficulties, job dissatisfaction, poor performance in chosen career, financial difficulties, conflict between career and family goals, and the age thirty transition.

Later in adulthood, from age 35 to 50, women's concerns and tasks center on reworking previous developmental issues and confronting new issues and challenges. A woman may evaluate her accomplishments in personal and professional areas. A crisis may arise from awareness of physical decline, chronic illness in her and/or her spouse's children, rejection by adolescent children, decisions about caring for an elderly parent, death or prolonged illness of parents, career setbacks, conflicts at work, financial concerns, moving associated with a job promotion, unemployment, sense of discrepancy between life goals and achievements, dissatisfaction with goals achieved, regret over past decisions related to marriage and having children, marital problems, return to work after raising children, and death of friends.

During the mature stage, concerns of women older than 50 center on consolidating their experiences and resources and reorienting one's life toward later years.

Chapter 3: Common Triggers & How To

Avoid Them

If you want to treat your anxiety successfully, you will want to understand what triggers it. Some people confuse the underlying cause of anxiety with the triggers, so it is best to define them up front. Whatever caused your anxiety disorder is something that you cannot avoid or change. It is the event, or series of events, that led to you getting this disorder. A trigger is much different. A trigger is a specific action or event that triggers an attack, or an outbreak of anxiety, in whatever form you happen to have the condition in.

Each of the types of anxiety disorder listed in the previous chapter have specific triggers. Although these triggers are a little bit different for each person that has the disorder, they are remarkable similar in the category or type of disorder itself. They can each be grouped into a specific type of event that triggers that type of anxiety. For example, undesired thoughts can trigger an episode of obsessive compulsive disorder while the trigger for panic disorders are often physical sensations.

It is vital that you understand your particular disorder clearly and what triggers it. Knowing what your personal triggers are can help you to minimize the number of anxiety attacks that you have. Some of these triggers are environmental, and you probably know what they are. For example, having an extremely stressful job or being in a relationship that causes a great deal of stress can both trigger anxiety. Anytime you have long term stress that remains consistent, you have a recipe for anxiety attacks.

Some Other Triggers of Anxiety

Thinking: People that don't stay busy may find that they have racing thoughts that they cannot control which turn into a problem. Those that have too much alone time with their thoughts will find that eventually those thoughts may trigger an anxiety attack. It is an endless circle once the process starts, because the anxiety may cause thoughts to become more negative, while the thoughts themselves create more anxiety.

Lack of Goals: One of the most important things that you can do to prepare yourself for a life free of anxiety is to make sure that you are always working towards something. Setting goals for yourself and working towards them will give your mind something to focus on, and it will allow you to keep those anxious thoughts from taking over. Even more importantly, when you reach those goals, you have reinforced a very positive feeling that will help you cope with anxiety in the future.

The Media: The media can be a major trigger factor when it comes to anxiety. The reason for this is quite simple – the media reports are very negative in nature. The media offers stories about young people dying, violent deaths and major disasters. These all can cause anxiety and paranoia among those who have an anxiety disorder.

Replacement Coping: This is a very common problem among those who have anxiety problems. They will replace any coping mechanisms that they have created with a much easier way to deal with thoughts – most commonly with drugs and alcohol. Those that use these replacements to deal with stress find that these negative behaviors are ultimately destructive, and eventually, those people will lose their natural or created mechanisms for coping.

Panic Attack Triggers

Panic attacks have their own set of triggers. Panic attacks are pretty rare, but for those who experience them, even the simple act of thinking about their panic attacks, and dreading them, can cause the attack to occur. Generally, people will get a panic attack when they are under stress, but more commonly, people will feel fear or dread about a certain feeling or sensation that they experience and this hypersensitivity to physical sensations will lead to a panic attack. However, there are some physical markers that you can look out for that may give you a clue that a panic attack is coming, and therefore take steps to prevent it.

Chest pains or feelings of tightness

Lightheadedness or dizziness

Irregular heartbeat or rapid heartbeat

Trouble taking deep breaths

Fears about your health, and thoughts of doom or dread.

Chapter 4: Types Of Meditation

Meditation is a broad topic that encompasses different practices, it isn't just about the chanting, counting the beads in a rosary, breathing, listening to a repetitive gong, staring at a candle flame, or sitting cross-legged in an empty room. It is about attaining relaxation where you enter into a restful state of mind that is beyond any conscious thinking where nothing around you really matters but what is going on in your mind. How you get there doesn't really matter, the most important thing is that you can attain pure consciousness irrespective of your posture. The proponents of meditation have come to a consensus that the best way to attain the needed relaxation to enter into the pure consciousness state is through practicing different meditation techniques some of which are outlined here:

Concentration Meditation

This entails putting all your focus on a single point, it could be repeating a single word, staring at a candle flame, counting beads on a rosary or listening to a repetitive gong to help capture your mind's attention hence ensuring that it doesn't wander away. With this meditation technique, you can isolate the random thoughts making it easy to move directly to the space within the many thoughts where pure consciousness exists. Given that this requires good concentration skills, attaining meditation using this technique is a sure way of improving your concentration.

Mindfulness Meditation

With this type of meditation, you grow to increase your awareness and acceptance through being mindful of the present moment that you are living. It entails broadening your conscious awareness where you focus on what you are experiencing at the time of the meditation, it could be the flow of your breath, your heartbeat and other rhythmic movements. All you have to do is observe the thoughts or emotions and let each one of them to just pass without judging them if you want to continue being in the "empty mind".

Guided meditation/visualization or guided imagery

You can also go through meditation through the help of a guide or teacher whereby you go through a process of experiencing a state of relaxed mind through engaging all your senses. The use of all the senses helps you form mental images of situations or places to help you attain a state of mental relaxation.

Yoga

This entails engaging in a series of controlled breathing routines and postures to help attain a state of relaxed or calm mind. It focuses on poses that push you to concentrate in order to attain the right balance hence enabling you to forget about whatever could be troubling you for some time as you try to balance and attain the needed concentration to do various poses. You can thus attain a state of being naturally present with continuous yoga poses.

Tai Chi

Entails doing various physical routines in a slow manner while controlling your breathing to attain a deep sense of calmness. It is one of the gentle forms of Chinese martial arts.

Transcendental Meditation

This technique involves allowing your mind to be in a state of being settled inwardly through the quieter levels of thought where you get to experience your inner self at the most peaceful/quiet level of self-awareness. It allows us to experience our innermost calmness, a state of our least excitation without chanting or focusing on our breath. It is where you attain a restful state of mind without actually thinking, your mind is actually empty when you are doing transcendental meditation.

Walking Meditation

With waking meditation, you walk without necessarily going anywhere, all you have to do is walk at a slow/medium pace then try to focus on what happens to your feet as you walk. You will find yourself in the space between your thoughts where you feel calm and relaxed irrespective of what you are going through.

Qi Gong Meditation

This entails combining physical movement with relaxation, breathing and balance exercises and meditation to attain calmness in the midst of all the thoughts going on in your mind at a certain time.

Gratitude Exercises

These entail focusing on things that matter to you most such as your loved ones whereby you look for what you like most about them then say a word of gratitude to them in your mind. This is best done when you wake up, preferably the first thing you think of when you wake up before thinking of other things like what you are going to wear or how the day will be hectic.

You can choose any meditation technique based on your personal preferences. Other specialized meditation techniques exist for many other situations including but not limited to meditation for insomnia, chi kung, meditation for easing menopause symptoms and many other forms of specialized meditation.

Chapter 5: Dealing With Separation

Anxiety

Identifying the most applicable treatment and remedy to your anxiety problem entails identifying the type of anxiety disorder you might have developed through the years. Many people spend their lives suffering from long-term symptoms of their harmful conditions without seeking professional help and support from family and friends who understand the situation. That will all change right now, starting with you facing your disorder head-on.

Separation Anxiety

This is a common anxiety problem in children. It is normal for kids to get scared, cry, throw tantrums and feel clinginess to people they care about, mostly with parents. However, when that anxiety does not go away through the years, it hinders the social development of the child, affecting both child and parent. In the long run, it will interfere with relationships and mental development.

Although separation anxiety will go away on most kids, some of them carry the condition until adulthood, creating anti-social behaviors. In adults, separation anxiety can breed obsession, which needless to say, leads to selfishness, jealousy and ultimately, wrath.

For children, the most common symptoms are worries and fears, while in adults, it can manifest physical symptoms. A person with separation anxiety will do anything and reason out anything just to stay at home, out of the limelight, within the sight of the person being clung to. There might also be an intense fear that something bad will happen to the person affected or the person being clung to should separation happen. Many kids also fear permanent separation, most likely due to a traumatic experience in the earlier years.

On advance cases, headaches and stomachaches are also seen in children, which later on can aggravate to chronic depression.

What are the best ways to handle separation anxiety?

Patience – If you have a family member with this disorder, keep having patience and just try to build his/her independence and confidence by encouragement. Being "anxious" about your family's anxiety disorder will just make matters worse.

Practice separation – -Do not force total separation. The process is slow and cannot be hasten because a kid with separation anxiety senses coercion, which signals him/her that there is something wrong.

Try pushing your kid to a crowd of other children or in the care of teachers or caregivers without leaving his/her sight. Just keep a distance but stay where he/she can see you for reassurance. This will develop social skills, which will make its way to his/her mind, covering anxiety disorder on its own.

Schedule separation after enforcing positive mood – What is a positive mood?

This is when the child is emotionally stable or has positive emotions, such as after eating, after resting, while playing, while being entertained or after receiving a reward. This will reduce panic attack, making it more manageable.

Have a goodbye ritual – For some people, a goodbye ritual can be a reassurance that the separation is not final. For some, it means non-verbal encouragement to stay brave against all the fears in the head. It can be as simple as a goodbye kiss, a wave, a special handshake or chant.

Develop familiarity – You cannot just bring a kid with separation anxiety to a school then expect him/her to behave and stay calm. Using the element of "shock" will make the fear worse. Why don't you just bring in a tutor, nanny or other kids to your house so your kid can develop familiarity and assurance that mingling with other people is not bad to begin with?

Don't stall when leaving – Stalling reinforces fear. If you will say you have to go, preferably after your goodbye ritual, just go. The kid will sense your hesitation, and as adults know, hesitation means there is something wrong.

Never scare an anxious kid – Some parents would say *"Do this or I will leave you"* or *"If you do that, I will leave you"* just make their kids follow them. However, this installs fear that a kid might carry until his/her grown up years. Letting a kid watch scary shows and movies will also reinforce fear in his mind – not a good move if you are trying to train independence.

Listen – This is the most recommended move for a child who already manifests isolation. Listen to what the child has to say. Do what he/she wants so the kid will do the same with you.

Never try cold shoulder treatment – It is easy to lose patience on a kid with unmanageable tantrum. Talking even if its is hard will pay off sooner of later, but giving the silence or cold treatment will make him/her harbor negative thoughts and emotions – the last thing you want to happen.

Chapter 6: Identifying The Physical, Emotional And Behavioral Manifestations Of Anxiety

Anxiety often comes about as a result of deep, unresolved emotional issues. But despite it being an emotional and mental problem, anxiety can often be detected and seen by way of its physical, emotional and behavioral manifestations.

Some of the physical manifestations of anxiety include the following:

1) You experience a surge of adrenaline as a result of the fact that you are always up on your toes.

2) Worrying and fearfulness are usually accompanied by any or a combination of the following: difficulty in breathing, dizziness, ringing in the ears, rapid heart rate, inability to talk properly, involuntary trembling, muscle tension, stiffness and profuse sweating.

3) You harbor an inability to sleep at night. This insomnia is caused in large part by

your constant fears and your inability to relax.

4) You experience sudden weight loss or weight gain. When you are afraid or worried, you tend to either overeat or eat little to nothing at all. This is what causes the abrupt change in weight.

5) When you are afraid, the body secretes stress hormones. The body is normally able to deal with these hormones only if they appear in long intervals. If you are a chronic worrier, then this also causes a constant stream of stress hormones in the body, which could eventually suffer from illnesses such as weakening of the immune system, cardiovascular disorders and digestive problems.

Some of the emotional manifestations of anxiety include the following:

1) You have a tendency to overestimate your fears and underestimate your ability to come to terms with such fears.

2) You suffer from mood swings.

3) You harbor a constant fear of getting caught unaware, or of either failing or disappointing the people around you.

4) Due to your negative thought patterns, you choose to dwell on the negative stuff instead of paying attention to the positives.

Some of the behavioral manifestations of anxiety include the following:

1) You harbor a strong desire to escape or avoid your anxiety triggers.

2) You suffer from irritability or the tendency to easily flip out, even on trivial matters.

3) You develop paranoia.

4) You experience sudden episodes of crying.

5) You experience wild outbursts.

6) You have a constant need to be reassured that everything will be alright.

The next chapter deals with the various risk factors and triggers that exacerbate your anxiety, as well as the debilitating effects that those who are afflicted with this condition are likely to experience.

Chapter 7: Recognizing Social Anxiety And

Social Phobia

As we mentioned in the previous chapter, there are some subtle ways of distinguishing between a person who is shy and introverted and a person who suffers from social phobia.

The problem, however, is that the person who is actually experiencing social anxiety disorder seldom realizes the problem themselves. This disorder is something they have been familiar with for a long time, perhaps all their life. As a child, they have seen the same traits in their parents - the social aloofness, the uncomfortable interactions with outsiders - and this is what they consider to be normal behavior. Therefore, it is actually difficult for them to understand that their aversion to social dealings is actually not ordinary, but a problem on their part.

Thus, it is usually someone within a close proximity to a socially anxious person who first notices the symptoms, usually someone who spends a lot of time with them. This person may know them in a personal manner, and may be someone such as a spouse, sibling, close friend, colleague, or even offspring and parents in some cases.

If you have an inclination that someone close to you is not 'just shy or awkward', but has moderate to acute social anxiety disorder, there are a few ways for you to be sure.

Natural shyness apart, there are a few day-to-day activities that may be ordinary to a person, but extremely difficult for a person experiencing social phobia. These are activities as simple as the following:

Making a phone call to strangers

Making a phone call in public

Making small talk at a gathering

Being watched while doing something

Being teased, even in a playful manner, by friends or family

Ordering food at a restaurant

Calling a server or a waiter at a restaurant

Being approached by a stranger

Approaching a stranger to be introduced

Approaching a stranger for information or help

Being called on in class or in a meeting

Being asked a question in public

Asking someone out on a date

Going on a date with someone and making conversations with them

Using bathrooms in public or in someone else's house

Working in front of others

Eating or drinking in front of others

Taking exams

Asking questions in class

As well as in some generally nervous situations, such as,

Speaking in public

Performing on stage

Being the center of attention

Most people who experience social anxiety disorder will show some specific reactions when facing these situations. These reactions and behaviors are divided into three groups of symptoms.

Emotional Symptoms

Intense Anxiety

Becoming self-conscious

Afraid of being judged or criticized by others

Fear of being ridiculed and humiliated

Intense worrying for days or weeks

Fear of embarrassing themselves with their actions

Fear that others would know that they are anxious

Fear that people will be embarrassed by them

Physical Symptoms

Intense blushing

Breathlessness, or shortness of breath

Excessive sweating

Nausea, i.e. vomiting

Shaky voice

Hot flashes

Frequent heartbeat or heart palpitations

Muscle tension

Cold and clammy hands

Diarrhea or upset stomach

Feeling faint, dizziness

Trembling or feeling wobbly

Behavioral Symptoms

Feeling confused about how to act

Avoiding social situations even at a great expense

Always remaining quiet

Hiding in the background at a gathering

Suddenly leaving or disappearing from a gathering

Always bringing someone else to social functions

Unwilling to meet new people

Avoiding eye contact while making conversation

Failing to ask questions or answer queries of strangers at a gathering

Not talking unless absolutely necessary

Avoiding crowds and preferring to blend into the surroundings

Avoiding situations where they might be the center of attention

Avoiding doing things that will need them to communicate with others, such as asking for food or the location of the toilet

There are a number of Social Anxiety tests available to screen the level of a person's phobia of society, especially if someone wants to test themselves. These tests are available everywhere, in medical institutions, research centers and online. We have prepared a questionnaire for you to test yourself, or a person close to you who you feel might have social anxiety disorder. If you think that you or they might need professional help, just fill out the form and take a print out to your doctor.

1. Do you feel troubled -

that people may be judging you?

that people may not like you?

when you are required to have an one-to-one conversation with a stranger?

by the thought of speaking in public?

by the idea of going to a social gathering alone?

2. Are you constantly worried -

that you will make mistakes in front of people?

that you would look foolish and stupid in front of others?

that people will find you boring and irritating?

that you will be humiliated and ridiculed by others?

that people would know that you are tensed and nervous?

3. While at a social gathering, do you -

prefer to blend in with the background?

stay quiet until someone speaks to you?

avoid talking to people you don't know?

increase your drinking to make the time easier to pass?

go to great lengths to avoid people who may want to speak to you?

avoid certain actions because you may require to ask someone's help?

intend to stay as less as you can?

fear that you may at one time become the center of attention?

feel worried that you may need to talk to someone you don't know?

4. Do you, more often than not -

feel worthless and insignificant?

feel disinterested in living?

feel depressed and gloomy?

feel tensed and nervous?

feel self-conscious around people?

feel that your fears are irrational and unreasonable?

5. Does your 'symptoms' -

interfere with our daily life activities?

led to a change in your eating habits?

led to an increase or decrease in your sleep?

led to an increase in your drinking or smoking?

led you to try any drugs?

induced any thoughts of suicide or harming yourself?

If you feel that you or a close family member/friend is experiencing social phobia, then most of these questions would seem very familiar to you. If you answered, "YES" to most of these questions, it is quite possible that you are suffering from Acute Social Anxiety Disorder, and you should seek out help as soon as possible.

Chapter 8: Managing Stress

Stress is the sensation of being overwhelmed by responsibilities or pressure. As a psychological concept, stress was first introduced in the 1950's, with the term originally taken from physics, where it described the amount of tension placed upon an object.

The important part of the stress definition is **feeling overwhelmed.** Many people have huge levels of responsibility but nonetheless thrive in difficult or taxing situations. Stress is the distinct feeling of being pushed or pulled too thin and it doesn't directly correlate to the level of responsibility that you may have, although responsibility and pressure are often factors.

Stress has a huge range of symptoms. It is known that it can increase blood pressure and heart rate, affect sleeping patterns, produce a loss of appetite, destroy concentration and contribute to a wide range of mental illnesses, such as depression.

When a person feels a sensation of stress, the body's hormonal system kicks into action. The nervous system releases a cocktail of hormones, most notably cortisol, which collectively trigger the 'flight or fight' response.

To simplify, the flight or fight response is an evolution adaptation that prepares the body to either combat a threat ('fight') or run away ('flight'). Ultimately this causes the heart rate to increase, the breath to become faster as well as a redirection of blood flow towards the muscles. More severe effects include shaking, loss of peripheral vision and the constriction of blood vessels. All of these responses are intended to prime the body for dealing with threats or challenges.

Whilst the fight or flight system is a fantastic adaptation that helped our ancestors cope with a harsh and dangerous world, it causes us a range of problems in modern society.

The vast majority of us are not going to need to fight to the death or run away from an apex predator when we experience a stressor. Rather our challenges are commonplace but chronic; a lack of money, workplace issues, interpersonal relationship strains, other desires and aspirations, etc.

The issue is that our flight and fight response can trigger in reaction to these mundane, but non-life threatening issues. If this response triggers too frequently, a high amount of flight & fight hormones are released, especially cortisol, into the body, producing the psychological sensation of stress.

Once you begin to understand that stress is a **response**, the methods in which stress can be tackled start to become clear – recognize what is causing the stress response and manage that.

Anything that causes a stress response is called a **stressor.** The crucial part of stressors is that they can be divided into

physiological stressors and **psychological** stressors.

Physiological stressors are events that directly put pressure upon the body, such as injury or extreme environmental temperatures.

Psychological stressors, however, are any events that are **perceived** as threatening or challenging. Depending upon the individual, this may include genuinely dangerous events (such as being mugged or attacked) to events that are actually harmless (such as an offhand comment interpreted negatively).

Therefore to manage stress, you need to analyze both your proximity to stressors and your perception of them. It may be the case that you have too many stressors within your life, in which case you need to cut back on events that are causing you stress.

However, it may be that you are interpreting too many manageable events as stressors, in which case you need to alter the ways you are perceiving these events.

Additionally, stress can also be managed by adopting a healthier lifestyle, which can manage the physiological causes and symptoms of stress. Let us walk through each of these solutions to stress in turn.

Chapter 9: Socially Scared Is Common

Social anxiety is one of the most common fears human beings have. Everyone has anxiety about being social but some people can't deal with the emotions that come with being around a social environment. Some people can't even handle going down the street and buying groceries because they are so insecure about social situations. I have no judgement for people that are in this position because I used to be that person. I used to not be able to go out without feeling tremendous levels of anxiety.

It's a sad way of living but it takes a lot of effort and courage to break yourself out of those places. When I was a teenager I was coping through life and not living it to the fullest. You can't live life to the fullest if you can't handle being social because it's a big part of growing. Communicating with people around you is part of life and we are in the age where technology is growing rapidly and we communicate through it.

The problem is these days most people are so insecure because they aren't communicating face to face and talking through a computer or a phone. I used to have a job years ago where I would sit behind a computer all day and I was happy with that because I didn't have to talk to anyone because that's what I feared the most. I used to be more driven because I wanted a job that I didn't have to go in a see people every day.

It wasn't until I got a wakeup call that I wasn't feeling happy and my anxiety got to the point where I couldn't handle it. I saw the future and was scared more about going through my entire life and not living it. I think we all think about the future but we don't really take time to look at the consequences where our actions are taking us. We get stuck coping through our pain and getting through the day instead of thriving with positive emotions. I wrote this book because that's what my job is, it's helping teens especially get through social anxiety so they can live their dreams. Been doing this for 10years now and the reward I get is a sense of freedom every day.

The reason I followed this path was because I know exactly what it feels like to cope through life and watch other people live it right in front of you. You see a version of yourself like you could do that too but you are controlled by your beliefs and have so many rules on what's appropriate. I used to love the movie fight club because I could relate so much with the character. It was about a man who lives a boring life and doesn't want to associate with anyone and just lets life go by without living. He hallucinates a guy who is everything he wants to be. Good looking, driven, successful, confident and loves uncertainty.

His name is Tyler Durden. He hallucinates the version of himself that just lets go of everything that holds him back. This movie literally made me cry when I first saw it because that is what I used to do every day. I used to visualize myself doing all these crazy things that I thought were incredibly brave, but in reality it was just a dream. Most people get caught up doing that aswell and they just numb their pain through watching reality tv shows.

Game of Thrones is the latest TV show out and everyone watches that. I know a good friend that has watched all the episodes 4times over. He has really bad social anxiety but his head is caught up in TV show world and you wonder why he feels not confident about life. I'm going to help you break out of the chains that you have put around yourself and it's actually not your fault. You have been conditioned by society to feel insecure and not feel comfortable putting your real self out there. We are taught to just be told how to feel and just don't break out of what you're doing. The people that you perceive to be the most confident people started where you were but just found the courage to stop worrying about what other people think of them.

How can you really have a good life if you care what people think. You can't and that's the truth because if you have social anxiety you wouldn't feel much happiness at all. You don't often see someone who is the happiest person in the world but has extreme social anxiety, you don't see it. It's a prison that you are in and there are ways to get yourself out of it and start living your purpose.

To break out of the position you are in you will need to change your identity and I know that sounds big. If you don't expand your identity and turn it into a new person everything in your life will stay the same. I don't mean you're going to have to change everything in your life but definitely have to shake your life up. Your nervous system is conditioned a certain way and it's been conditioned by your daily habits. If you change your day up, your nervous system will go into a shock and that point is where we make progress. I made a decision years ago that I was going to change everything in my life no matter how scary it seemed and I was certain this was going to happen.

I was motivated some days to change but other days I just wanted to stay at home and give up. This process is a hard one but worth it because you will feel the most alive you ever have. I didn't realize but when we feel an emotion that's when we are the most alive. When you sit at home all day and maybe feel depressed and anxious you get addicted to those emotions so it feels comfortable for you. When you step out regular patterns and your comfort zone you will feel alive and awake.

That's honestly what people want more than anything. We think we want a new house or something external but what we really want is some core emotional feelings. When we are coping we are at the lowest of our emotion and it's hard to grow from that place. When we break out of a success barrier we become our real self but it's scary to do. Let me ask you a simple question, are you fulfilled everyday living the life your living? Are you a bit scared of expressing yourself to the fullest? When I ask people this question they can rationalize that it's fine when it's not.

A big key to experience a shift is to tell yourself the truth and be real. You can lie to yourself and act like you have it all together because you know deep down its fake. When was the last time you really looked and felt how you have been living and got emotional about it? This is what happened to me and knowing I was going to be like this in the future scared me. Can you imagine living with bad anxiety and being afraid of living for another five years, at some point there has to be a defining moment that changes everything and I want that moment to be right now for you.

Time is the most valuable thing we have and sitting here wasting it & feeling sorry for yourself won't help you in anyway. You can sit there hoping someday a miracle is going to happen or you can realize that you're the only person keeping yourself stuck. Another big thing people who have anxiety do is they try and cheat the system. What I mean exactly is they look for instant gratification like drugs, alchohol, anti-depressants and ways of not being in control. They are relying on some stimulus to change the way they feel and by doing this in the long run it destroys your life. I have had a good friend who had bad social anxiety and depression and she was on anti-depressants for years.

She told me she used to feel like she was numb and still had bad depression and anxiety. It doesn't matter what kind of drug you take if you are still talking to yourself in a negative way on a consistent basis then you will still feel stressed out. Do you talk to yourself in a positive way on a regular basis or do you beat yourself up often? One of the big distinctions that changed my life in 2012 was we are the only person that abuses ourselves.

Most people blame their circumstances on other people or some event so it takes the focus off themselves but if you have anxiety right now it's your own fault. This is a hard pill to swallow but everyone I have told this to knows it the truth deep down but they don't want to admit it to themselves. I could tell you that I know the secret for you to never feeling anxiety again but that would be completely false. Anxiety is a good emotion as long as it's a counsellor and not a jailer.

If any book you read says they know the secret to never feeling anxiety again it's just a marketing strategy but there are ways you can be able to handle it so it doesn't control your life. When significant emotional experiences happen that we can't control, of course we are going to be feeling anxious and scared because it's uncertainty. Anything we do that is uncertain is going to make us feel anxious. If I asked a person with social anxiety to just go walk up to a stranger and make a conversation, straight away it would produce fear in this person. Even though they haven't done it yet you see. We can feel anxious about things that haven't happened yet but we play them out in our heads like they have. I have worked with people with social anxiety and it's not the action that scares them but the thought. You get certain pictures in your head about what's going to happen and you are certain about it.

One thing I am certain about is that we blow things way out of proportion in our heads and that's what makes us so scared. If you go out of your house and socialise with people what's the worst thing that's going to happen? Most people tell me that someone might yell at them, reject them or make them feel embarrassed. So what we are scared about is those feelings but what you didn't realize is you get to determine what your experiences means to you. Two people can have the exact same experience and you might feel anxious & embarrassed about it and I could feel euphoric, perception is everything.

I want to give you a little teaching on perception that will blow you mind. Whoever you think you are in the moment that's your reality and that's who you are. You could be the most confident person in the world if you bought into that reality but most people don't think things can shift that fast. Haven't you had times in your life where you have been excited and felt like you could conquer the world? Of course you have but most people only experience that once every so often and just hope those times will happen.

The only way you will experience those times more is to expand your identity and challenge yourself and use your willpower to do it. How many times a day do you see opportunities that you know you should be taking but you hold back? You have heard the quote that your life starts at the end of your comfort zone and that's the truth. The comfort zone is something that you should love experiencing and if you challenge yourself with this all your anxiety and fears will go away.

A big reason why people have massive social anxiety is because they have friends that make them feel that way. I have seen people who have friends that constantly put them down and they do it like a habit. We don't know how insecure people are and they might be good at hiding it but some people take words to heart and let it destroy them. I have talked to people that have said, 'this happened to me in my past' or 'this person said I'm ugly.'

Are you really going to let someone else's opinion of you become your reality and everything you think about? Are you going to be on your death bed later in life and be thinking about what someone said to you or do you need a wakeup call right now. I tell people to wake up and start feeding them positivity because we are either feeling love in the moment or fear. You can say to yourself that you are amazing and you're confident but most people would rather indulge in how they can't help themselves. Realize everyone in this world has social anxiety, it's part of being human but some people can change from coping with it to thriving.

Chapter 10: What Type Are You?

• Do you want the support of others or are you a Greta Garbo, "I want to be alone" type? Meditation or progressive muscle relaxation will recharge your batteries and quiet your mind while giving you the solitude you crave.

• Are you an A type personality? A class setting will give you the social interaction, stimulation, motivation and support you're looking for.

Consult with your doctor first if you have a history of muscle spasms, back problems, or other serious injuries that may be aggravated by tensing muscles.

• Get comfortable by taking off shoes and loosening clothing.

• Breath in and out in slow, deep breaths for a few minutes to relax.

• Ready to go? Relaxed, look at right foot. Focus for a moment on how it feels.

• Holding for ten seconds, lowly tense the muscles as tightly as you can in your right foot.

• Now relax that foot. Tension should be flowing away, so focus on the way your foot feels as it becomes loose and limp.

• Breathe slowly and deeply for a moment while you stay in this relaxed state.

• Shift attention to your other foot when ready. Duplicate your actions.

• Contract and relax each muscle group as you move slowly up your body.

• Try not to tense muscles other than what you are focused on - it may take practice.

Chapter 11: Detox, How To Remove The

Physical Causes Of Anxiety

Without further ado, let's dive right in to how to conquer your anxiety. The first tool which we are going to use is to change the diet, we are going to go on a detox. The reason this is the first step in beating your anxiety isn't because it is the most interesting or exciting, it is because it is *necessary for any other tip to work!*

So many books start with the positive thinking aspect of beating anxiety but ignore your diet and the role it plays in your mood. When I was very anxious I was taking a pre-workout (energy drink) every day before I went to the gym. As soon as I stopped drinking this I noticed my anxiety got significantly better and I knew that the diet is strongly related to how you feel. The following detox diet will be very helpful to you to reduce some of the more acute symptoms of anxiety before we do the more challenging exercises

Get rid of the caffeine

I am a recovering coffee addict. I love the stuff, the smell, the taste, the warm cup in my hand, everything. I especially love the massive surge in motivation I get after a nice large pot of coffee.

I used to drink between 3 and 4 French press pots of coffee per day, for those of you keeping score that is about 10 cups. It is now wonder I was anxious constantly!

This girl seems to have had a similar experience.

https://www.psychologytoday.com/blog/progress-not-perfection/201106/i-quit-coffee-cure-my-anxiety

The interesting thing about caffeine is that when it goes into your body, it actually stimulates your adrenal glands (on top of your kidneys) which end up dumping epinephrine (adrenaline) into your bloodstream. You know what else stimulates these glands? Getting in a fight or being chased by a lion!

By drinking caffeine you are artificially putting your body into a fear response. This is useful fuel for getting things done if you drink just enough coffee to kick off a small stress and fear response, (about one small cup) but most of us drink it by the jug full. Our culture (and particularly the culture where I live, Seattle, home of Starbucks) works coffee into every occasion and caffeine into every beverage.

Waking up? Drink a coffee.

Going on a date? Make it a coffee date.

Going to the gym? Have an energy drink.

Want a soda? It's loaded with caffeine

...You get the picture.

If you are serious about overcoming your anxiety, cut caffeine out of your diet *completely.* After you have done that then you can slowly reintroduce it and find a happy medium.

Pro-tip* If you are suffering from caffeine withdrawals you can switch from coffee and energy drinks to green tea and from there go cold turkey. Baby step it, just make sure you get off of it.

Eat tons of fat

Eating omega 3 fatty acids is good for the brain. It reduces inflammation and daily wear and tear which goes on in the brain, that's why mom always called salmon brain food.

If you are worried about getting fat from eating fat, don't worry! That has been proven to be BS (Bad Science) eating good fats doesn't make you fat (I eat more fat in a day than most people in a week and am doing fine).

If you are wondering where to find all the fat that you are going to need in your diet then here a few sources:

Nuts and nut butters

Whole milk and or cream

Avocados

Salmon

Coconut oil

Find a way to work those into your diet daily and you will notice a boost in your mood.

*Pro-tip, here is a great recipe for salmon encrusted in walnuts, a 2 for 1 (maybe slice an avocado over it too?)

http://thehealthyfoodie.com/maple-walnut-crusted-salmon/

Drink tons of water

The body is kind of like a pool, if you don't have water moving through it tends to turn green and slimy inside.

All jokes aside, drinking lots of water is one of the top things you can do for your health and for boosting your mood. The body is always making stress hormones and for those of us suffering from anxiety it is making more than normal.

Drinking lots of water helps flush out the toxins in the body more efficiently. So here is your action step, if you are a big guy like me (200+pounds) then drink a gallon of water a day, not Gatorade, not juice, water.

If you are smaller person drink somewhere between a half gallon and a full gallon per day.

Supplement magnesium

Yes, this tip is going to cost a little money but trust me, it is worth it, Magnesium plays a key role in all of our bodies reactions and it is something which is very deficient in our modern diet. Our soils and as a result our food is deficient in magnesium and our water is filtered by the state to have less magnesium, so you and I have to supplement it.

Studies have shown that a magnesium drastically reduces feelings of stress, anxiety, and depression

https://www.psychologytoday.com/blog/evolutionary-psychiatry/201106/magnesium-and-the-brain-the-original-chill-pill

Try taking it as recommended on the bottle and see if your mood doesn't improve:

Chapter 12: Evidence-Based Analysis

Of course, no victory can be one without the help of evidence. One big element of always feeling anxious and scared comes from the fact we stop surveying the evidence. On the moments that we do look at it, we are quick to dismiss any information that it provides as hopeful thinking. This is the mind of an anxious person – to believe that the answers they need differ from everyone else's. I've been there, and it's a brutal feeling.

Instead of just agreeing with your own script for Armageddon, though, why not challenge it? Ask your anxious mind to show it's working!

Anxiety can come from precedence – we only need to see one similar scenario and that gives our anxiety all it needs as "proof". From dealing with legal issues to your own physical health, it's very easy for the anxious mind to start developing the story for us, creating the ever more believable version of events. Someone else was taken to court for that and ruined, so will you. Somebody else had a sore rib and it turned out to be a rare cancer, so will you.

The problem with an anxious mind is that it makes it so incredibly easy to just blow your fears out of all proportion. It becomes staggeringly easy to find yourself in these situations without even thinking about it. Before you know it, your hyperbolic, totally fictional turn of events is as close to the truth as anyone is likely to get.

This dangerous mindset is all about limiting your chances to meet your ambition. Do not let that happen. Instead, ask yourself how you would react if a friend or loved one had the same anxieties. When they told you what the precedent was, the precedent you are convincing yourself is the major problem, how would you react to them?

Would it be with the same utter fear and dread that you are reacting to now?

It helps to survey the way you have been dealing with your anxiety, as you might just find that the biggest obstacle to defeating it is yourself. The minute you start to convince yourself that your problem is cut and dried just because it happened to someone/something else is when you allow your anxiety to take over.

So, stand up to the issue – look at the evidence for yourself. What real evidence points to your anxiety being right?

Chapter 13: Bipolar Disorder Treatment

Options

Bipolar disorder may be a crippling mental ailment, but it is manageable. Do not lose hope if you have been diagnosed of having bipolar episodes, it is not the end of the world. With the help of certain medications and doing a couple of healthy lifestyle changes, you can significantly decrease the number of episodes you get and also reduce their intensity.

Medications for Bipolar Disorder

Once you have experienced more than two bipolar episodes, you are therefore required to take maintenance medications for the rest of your life, or for the long term at the very least. Fortunately, once your doctor has stabilized your mood swings using medications, you will be taking lower doses as time passes.

Lamotrigine and Lithium are two of the most prescribed, and most effective, medications that are prescribed for bipolar patients. Although these drugs can and will provide you with relief, they do have some side effects that you need to be aware of.

Lamotrigine

Lamictal (commercially-available Lamotrigine) is the most popular, FDA-approved maintenance medication for adults suffering from bipolar disorder. This drug can delay and decrease the intensity of the mood swings that accompany bipolar disorder, more specifically the bouts of extreme depression.

Lamictal's was originally meant to be a anti-convulsant, a form of medication that is meant to prevent or delay seizures when treating people with epilepsy. It was only recently that medical researchers found out that it has significant mood-altering and antidepressant effects that can be useful in treating bipolar disorder.

Side Effects of Lamotrigine (Lamictal)

Common side effects that come with the use of Lamictal include, but are not limited to:

•Headaches

•Diarrhea

•Blurry Vision and Dizziness

•Weird Dreams and Slight Hallucinations

In addition, around 3 out of 1000 people are allergic to Lamotrigine. If you find that you have developed a very itchy rash shortly after using Lamictal, you should discontinue using it and tell your doctor, because oftentimes they can be fatal.

Lithium

Lithium (available under the brand names Eskalith and Lithobid) has been used to treat bipolar disorder and depression for the longest time; it has actually been around for more than fifty years. Lithium was once only thought to minimize and decrease the instances of patients' manic episodes, but later it was found out that it can also be used to treat bipolar depression.

Lithium is used as a long-term or lifetime maintenance treatment for bipolar disorder. If you have started using lithium to manage the symptoms of your bipolar episodes you need to follow your doctor's advice and not stop the treatment on your own. Studies have shown that more than 90% of patients who went against the advice of their doctors and stopped taking lithium experienced relapse, and they are often much worse than before. Another drawback of stopping lithium use abruptly rather than gradually can decrease the effectiveness of the drug if you ever relapse and need to take it again to control your extreme mood swings.

Around 75% of patients who were prescribed with Lithium have been reported to experience side effects, albeit very minor ones that can be treated by lowering the dosage. It is not advisable for you to lower your dosage on your own once you experience side effects, you should always consult with your doctor first.

Here are some of the said side effects of taking Lithium:
- Abrupt Weight Gain
- Memory Problems
- Loss of Focus and Problem Concentrating
- Confusion and Mental Slowness
- Hair Loss
- Acne Breakouts
- Excessive Thirst and Cottonmouth
- Excessive Urination
- Blurry Vision and Dizziness
- Nausea, Vomiting, and/or Diarrhea
- Decreased Thyroid Functions (can be counteracted using hormone therapy)

Some of the more serious side effects include the weakening of bones in children and cause birth defects in 1 out of 1000 childbirths. Long term Lithium treatments can also impair liver and kidney function, which is why patients need to undergo blood tests every couple of months to inform their attending physicians if there are any serious repercussions that need to be dealt with.

If you are not keen with the idea of medication, you really do not have any choice at this point in time. You need to take your medication regularly if you want your bipolar episodes to stop; there are no ifs and buts about it. Hopefully, in the near future, scientific studies will be able to find a permanent cure for bipolar disorder, but as of right now, all you can do is take your prescription medicines and learn how to cope with what you are dealt with.

Chapter 14: Generalized Anxiety Disorder:

When Worry Gets Out Of Control

What Is GAD?

Occasional anxiety is a normal part of life. You might worry about things like health, money, or family problems. But people with generalized anxiety disorder (GAD) feel extremely worried or feel nervous about these and other things—even when there is little or no reason to worry about them. People with GAD find it difficult to control their anxiety and stay focused on daily tasks.

The good news is that GAD is treatable. Call your doctor to talk about your symptoms so that you can feel better.

What are the signs and symptoms of GAD?

GAD develops slowly. It often starts during the teen years or young adulthood. People with GAD may:

Worry very much about everyday things

Have trouble controlling their worries or feelings of nervousness

Know that they worry much more than they should

Feel restless and have trouble relaxing

Have a hard time concentrating

Be easily startled

Have trouble falling asleep or staying asleep

Feel easily tired or tired all the time

Have headaches, muscle aches, stomach aches, or unexplained pains

Have a hard time swallowing

Tremble or twitch

Be irritable or feel "on edge"

Sweat a lot, feel light-headed or out of breath

Have to go to the bathroom a lot

Children and teens with GAD often worry excessively about:

Their performance, such as in school or in sports

Catastrophes, such as earthquakes or war

Adults with GAD are often highly nervous about everyday circumstances, such as:

Job security or performance

Health

Finances

The health and well-being of their children

Being late

Completing household chores and other responsibilities

Both children and adults with GAD may experience physical symptoms that make it hard to function and that interfere with daily life.

Symptoms may get better or worse at different times, and they are often worse during times of stress, such as with a physical illness, during exams at school, or during a family or relationship conflict.

What causes GAD?

GAD sometimes runs in families, but no one knows for sure why some family members have it while others don't. Researchers have found that several parts of the brain, as well as biological processes, play a key role in fear and anxiety. By learning more about how the brain and body function in people with anxiety disorders, researchers may be able to create better treatments. Researchers are also looking for ways in which stress and environmental factors play a role.

How is GAD treated?

First, talk to your doctor about your symptoms. Your doctor should do an exam and ask you about your health history to make sure that an unrelated physical problem is not causing your symptoms. Your doctor may refer to you a mental health specialist, such as a psychiatrist or psychologist.

GAD is generally treated with psychotherapy, medication, or both. Talk with your doctor about the best treatment for you.

Psychotherapy

A type of psychotherapy called cognitive behavioral therapy (CBT) is especially useful for treating GAD. CBT teaches a person different ways of thinking, behaving, and reacting to situations that help him or her feel less anxious and worried.

Medication

Doctors may also prescribe medication to help treat GAD. Your doctor will work with you to find the best medication and dose for you. Different types of medication can be effective in GAD:

Selective serotonin reuptake inhibitors (SSRIs)

Serotonin-norepinephrine reuptake inhibitors (SNRIs)

Other serotonergic medication

Benzodiazepines

Doctors commonly use SSRIs and SNRIs to treat depression, but they are also helpful for the symptoms of GAD. They may take several weeks to start working. These medications may also cause side effects, such as headaches, nausea, or difficulty sleeping. These side effects are usually not severe for most people, especially if the dose starts off low and is increased slowly over time. **Talk to your doctor about any side effects that you have.**

Buspirone is another serotonergic medication that can be helpful in GAD. Buspirone needs to be taken continuously for several weeks for it to be fully effective.

Benzodiazepines, which are sedative medications, can also be used to manage severe forms of GAD. These medications are powerfully effective in rapidly decreasing anxiety, but they can cause tolerance and dependence if you use them continuously. Therefore, your doctor will only prescribe them for brief periods of time if you need them.

Don't give up on treatment too quickly. Both psychotherapy and medication can take some time to work. A healthy lifestyle can also help combat anxiety. Make sure to get enough sleep and exercise, eat a healthy diet, and turn to family and friends who you trust for support.

What is it like to have GAD?

"I was worried all the time and felt nervous. My family told me that there were no signs of problems, but I still felt upset. I dreaded going to work because I couldn't keep my mind focused. I was having trouble falling asleep at night and was irritated at my family all the time.

I saw my doctor and explained my constant worries. My doctor sent me to someone who knows about GAD. Now I am working with a counselor to cope better with my anxiety. I had to work hard, but I feel better. I'm glad I made that first call to my doctor."

Chapter 15: Signs And Symptoms

So, what are the most common symptoms of having either an intense phobia or a sign of anxiety? They both can be remarkably similar. It becomes quite hard to determine if you feel anxious because of a phobia, or if you have the phobia because of being anxious all the time. The main issue that you want to look into, though, comes from understanding the major signs and symptoms.

Just remember that for many people, though, signs and symptoms that are associated with phobia and/or anxiety can differ. These are not universal; having them does not confirm anxiety/phobia, nor does not having these symptoms a clear indicator that everything's going fine.

The Major Signs

So, what stands out as the major issues and symptoms?

Excessive Sweating. Excessive and serious sweating is one of the major issues that stands out clearest for all. Excessive sweating is a major issue, one that can leave us feeling even more anxious around people. When you feel like you're sweating so much that people are taking notice it can be hard to just hide it all. However, if you are someone who does not feel too warm but seems to be producing a massive amount of sweat, you might be feeling anxious. You could even be suffering from a phobia you never knew about.

Trembling. A sense of trembling is rarer but can be seen in those who feel deeply anxious or are suffering from fear of phobia. The image of someone sweating heavily and trembling creates the image of someone who is quite ill. It can be quite distressing for people to see you like this, and thus trembling becomes a common problem that you need to find a way around. If you are trembling for no apparent reason, then you might be suffering from an anxious bout, or your phobias have kicked in.

Breathing Issues. Do you find that you are struggling to get a full inhale of air? Do you feel like when you take a deep breath, you get less than you should? It's not likely to be a blockage. People suffer from breathing issues but if it appears to come on when you are in the middle of a similar situation, it could be a phobia that causes you to feel anxious and worried when you are in certain events.

Tachycardia. A rapid and increasingly intense heartbeat can be the major problem that you have to deal with. Tachycardia is the sensation of feeling your heartbeat picking up pace to the point where it's actually quite off-putting for you.

Now, you could be suffering from one or two of these symptoms and it's not a point to the idea of anxiety or phobia. However, suffering from all? At once? It's about as clear an indication that you are dealing with an anxious state of mind.

You don't have to be actively suffering from a phobia to feel like this, though – it could be a life-related issue that is making you feel like this. To help you determine if that is the case, though, we recommend that you check the next section out.

There, we'll be looking at some of the most common signs and symptoms of suffering from typical anxiety.

Chapter 16: Treating Social Anxiety

Psychotherapy is the most common form of treating Social Anxiety. Cognitive Behavioral Therapy is the recommended form of Psychotherapy for those who are suffering from Social Anxiety Disorder and Panic Disorder. This treatment attends to dysfunctional emotions, and cognitive processes. It also addresses maladaptive behavior and thus is able to help those who are not flexible enough to adapt to certain situations and have a hard time dealing with life.

During Cognitive Behavioral Therapy, these things happen:

Psychological Assessment. This is an examination that determines the state of a person's mental health which in turn leads to the diagnosis of a mental ailment.

Conceptualization. In this stage, ways on how to treat a certain disorder are discussed based on the person's profile and on what he/she needs.

Skills Acquisition and Skills Training. Knowing a certain person's talents and skills will help that person develop confidence and will then help the person in developing his skills for the better. Knowing that you are able to do something and that you are capable of achieving something will help you in making yourself feel better and more accomplished.

Generalization. This is the assessment of a behavior and of a person's profile. Generalizing a disorder will then lead to being given certain medication that will help in fighting the said disorder.

Post-Treatment follow up. Of course, it is very important to know a person's progress after being given treatment or medication. Knowing how better a person has become or checking if that person really did become better will then help the doctor in knowing what else could be done or if the medications need to be stopped. It's a way of knowing if a person was able to respond to the medication or if that person got worse because of it.

Cognitive Behavioral Therapy is said to be very effective in the treatment of Social Anxiety and other anxiety disorders. The basic idea of CBT is that your thoughts and feeling play a huge role in your actions. So if one finds themselves thinking a lot about being embarrassed in front of people then they will avoid people and stay away from any situations that they could be embarrassed in. They try to teach that you cannot control the world around you but you can control how you think about things and how you control your emotions. A big part of this therapy is desensitization to stimules that triggers anxiety. Also this type of therapy is usually done in a group with people that have the same disorder and together they slowly progress step by step to help reduce their anxiety. It is best to do this as a group so you can have moral support along the way through your journey. A lot of the techniques in the next chapter touch on different parts of Cognitive Behavioral Therapy.

If you think you have Social Anxiety symptoms, then better check with a doctor and see what could be done. The earlier you get into therapy, the better.

Some adults have a hard time adapting with therapy because they cannot accept the fact that they have certain disorders that need to be treated. This is the reason why getting diagnosed early is very important.

However, if you are an adult and got diagnosed late in life, then it's no reason for you not to try your best to deal with therapy. Remember, if you want to live a good life, then you have to allow yourself to get help.

Chapter 17: What Is Anxiety Disorder?

Imagine this – you're strapped into a seat for a roller coaster ride. The car has just begun to move and is making its slow ascent to the top before it crashes down the rail in a topsy-turvy journey of excitement and exhilaration.

Feel the butterflies in the pit of your stomach building with every rail your car rides. As you reach the top, your heart begins to race, and you find that you're short of breath from the thrill you're expecting to begin at any moment.

Now, imagine that you're stuck on that track at the very top. There's a power fault which caused you to stall, and you don't know when the ride is going to continue, and as you wait for the roller-coaster to start again, your heart thuds and your palms become sweaty.

What if you were stuck at the top of that roller coaster for the rest of your life? What if that ride never resumed, and you were doomed to feel those butterflies, that agonising uncertainty and fear of 'what next', all your life.

Think of yourself at the grocery store, waiting in line to pay for your purchases, and feeling that fretfulness and worry in the pit of your stomach. Put yourself in a park, surrounded by little children running around you, and suffering bouts of fear and uneasiness, wondering if you've locked the door after you. Imagine yourself in the shower, and feeling an unreasonable fear that the water from the showerhead is going to drown you.

Now, imagine yourself living this intensified fear, this agonising worry, the uneasiness of feeling something is not right, every single day, and every single moment.

That is what people living with an anxiety disorder suffer from each day.

Generalised Anxiety Disorder is a disorder, a mental ailment – it is not something the sufferer brings upon themselves. The anxiety they feel is not an emotion that can be controlled. It is an endless suffering, of feeling that dread and uneasiness of being at the top of the roller coaster in everyday life.

A patient diagnosed with GAD does not really have a reason to feel anxious. It is a form of diffused anxiety which constantly hovers over the individual for no apparent reason. Unlike normal anxiety which results from an event such as waiting for an important exam result, GAD patients experience the terrible agony and worry without reason.

That is the most difficult stage of GAD, not having a reason for the terrible anxiety, for it means suffering the distress of worry and fear without an end. The simplest of tasks overwhelm the individual – getting up to make breakfast for the family, driving to work, or even sitting down for lunch with office colleagues. The day seems filled with worry and tension beyond their control.

The most common remark people suffering from anxiety disorders get to hear is to stop thinking about it. However, this disorder exists because the thought process cannot be stopped. Regardless of whether the individual is trying to function normally, working on lessening their anxiety, or having a full-blown anxiety attack, the thoughts run through their mind in a non-stop loop.

The most important thing to understand about anxiety is that it is beyond control. Anxiety Disorders are caused by external environmental factors, combined with the emotional well-being of the individual. This could be a simple factor, such as a change of workplace, moving to a different city, or even having a new baby.

Along with external factors, the genetic make-up, personality and the biological chemistry of the brain also matter when treating anxiety disorders. However, this does not mean that a sufferer is emotionally weak, or that they have a medical history of mental illnesses. Anxiety Disorders are triggered by a variety of factors, all coming together at the same time.

Anxiety, by itself, is not an enemy of the body. It acts as a warning signal to the body when danger is near. It prompts the body to prepare you to tune into the fight or flight mode. In a world where instinct and fear form a vital part of life's survival mechanism, anxiety is a very important emotion.

But it is when this emotion spills over in such a way that the worry and tension begin to occur without reason, or become exaggerated for reasons unknown, that it becomes a problem and is diagnosed as an Anxiety Disorder. So how do you differentiate between normal anxiety and an anxiety disorder?

Normal anxiety does not cause you to freeze during your daily activities; facing a cashier or taking a drink of water would not cause you to have irrational fears. The worry and tension that accompanies normal anxiety can be controlled, it is not something that takes over your day-to-day activities, overshadowing all other thoughts.

Normal anxiety also does not lead your worrying to reach extreme lengths that cause unnecessary stress to the body. A delayed reply to an email is just that, a delayed reply to an email. To someone suffering from GAD, a delayed reply would be a catastrophe leading to paranoia and terrible imaginings as to why the reply is delayed.

This is because normal anxiety is usually restricted to realistic scenarios, limited to situations which are probable. They are not diffused and irrational, existing for no reason. When you do feel anxiety, it would last only for a short while and subside when realised. On the other hand, GAD would cause the worry to be never-ending, stretching for months at a time in a continuous cycle of fear and worry, day in and out.

For a layman, trying to understand anxiety is very difficult. It is complicated to imagine not being able to stop feeling anxious. It seems difficult to grasp why someone would feel anxiety if they had no reason to actually be worrying.

So, what is anxiety disorder? To be better able to place yourself in a sufferer's shoes, and be empathetic to the problem they face, try to place yourself in the following scenarios:

- Imagine that you are sitting on a plane, and someone sitting in front of your seat takes something out of a bag in the overhead cabin. A small strap of the bag stays stuck in the door of the overhead cabin, hanging in the air. How would you react?

For a person suffering from anxiety, this could pose a very big issue. They would imagine that the strap would stop the cabin door from locking, and during turbulence, the heavy bags in the cabin could fall out and into someone's head, causing trauma or injury.

- If you have previously suffered from trauma, for instance, a car accident, then you would be able to have compassion for an individual who suffers intense anxiety because they fear the trauma recurring. The fear sets in the mind to such a crippling extent that it hampers their everyday life. A sufferer of PTSD caused by a car accident would feel severe anxiety about travelling in a car. Even getting into a car would be a cause for hyperventilation due to intense anxiety and fear.

PTSD is a form of phobia of the occurred trauma, combined with anxiety about having to do the task which caused the trauma. For a victim of a car accident, this would translate to an intense fear of travelling by cars, and anxiety about having to use cars in their everyday life.

- Imagine suffering from anxiety in your everyday life, but being unable to pinpoint why you're feeling so anxious. It is an uneasiness you feel in the pit of your stomach, a gnawing fear which makes your hands tremble, but there is nothing in your life that can cause you to worry in this manner.

Oftentimes, the anxiety faced by persons suffering from GAD is without reason. This is a form of diffused anxiety which continues to hover in a person's mind expressly because there is no reason for it to exist. It is an unwarranted fear in the individual's mind.

These are but a few examples of the problems people suffering from Anxiety Disorder face. The important thing to know is that this is a disorder that can be treated, both by modern medicine as well as techniques that can be applied at home. However, before we discuss how Anxiety Disorders can be treated, it is important to understand a different kind of anxieties that exist and to identify which type of anxiety the individual is suffering from.

In the next chapter, we will study the different forms of anxiety that exist.

Chapter 18: Symptoms Of Anxiety

Disorder And Panic Attacks

We have all experienced anxiety and panic attacks. Before you sit your driver's license test, or give a presentation to a large group, your heart is racing and hands are sweaty. We feel butterflies in our stomach before our first date. We worry over family problems or feel jumpy at the mere thought of asking the boss for a pay raise.

However, if worries and fears are stopping you from living your life to the full then you may be suffering from an anxiety disorder. There are great self-help management plans that can help you lessen your anxiety and panic attacks and take back control of your life.

It is normal to worry and feel tense or scared when under pressure or facing a stressful situation. Anxiety is the body's natural response to danger, an in built alarm that is set off when we feel there is a threat.

People who do not suffer from panic attacks may think that it is due to one's imagination. The fact is that for those who suffer from it, it is real and it has serious psychological and emotional effects on them. A panic attack can be so sudden and severe that the experience is the only symptom. The clinical term for these attacks is called Panic Anxiety Disorder.

Some people report that it can be triggered by a life-threatening situation that happens shortly just before the attack occurred. The person who suffers from the panic attacks may have some of the following symptoms and sensations:

Racing or pounding heart beat or palpitations - it's caused by increased adrenalin pumped into the body. Shortness of breath, difficulty in breathing or tightness in the chest - your chest feels as though it does not expand sufficiently to take in enough air

Shallow, rapid breathing with severe trembling, shaking fear or anxiousness - it is a normal reaction to fear

Feelings of nausea, light-headedness or dizziness can happen as blood flow is redirected from the gastrointestinal system - the increased adrenalin can cause distorted vision.

A feeling of dread is another reaction to fear as if something bad or terrible is going to happen soon.

A rapid pulse rate, sweating and a brief body temperature rise occur as the body is in a fight or flight state and perspiration is increased.

Some people even experience choking as the muscles in the throat constrict due to the anxiety which gives a feeling of choking or inability to swallow.

A feeling of intense chest pains as muscle tension is caused by the anxiety and it feels like a heart attack.

Some may experience hot flashes or chills - hot flashes are caused by the action of muscles tensing and releasing from the anxiety while chills are caused by the body cooling off the muscles through perspiration.

A sensation of tingling or numbness in the extremities in fingers or toes - the nervous system is confused from the activity occurring in the body and is sending false signals to all parts of the body.

A sense of losing control and fear because of the changes in levels of chemistry, the brain is confused and unsure of what is happening in the body, thus the impending 'insanity'.

The ultimate fear of death - the feelings of the anxiety are so intense and the physical manifestations of the disorder make the person feel as though they are going to die.

The above mentioned symptoms of anxiety and panic attacks can climax within a few minutes and hence, an initial episode will usually result in a trip to the emergency room.

Anxiety Disorder

This condition is when a person will build anxiety at a very quick rate causing it to build up and greatly increase stress levels until it finally releases in a temporary state of physical pain or discomfort known as a Panic attack.

Anxiety Disorder Symptoms

Avoidance

Confusion

Nervousness or very jumpy

Insecure or self-conscious

Frequently feeling restless or on edge

Feelings of dread, apprehension or uneasiness

Panic Attacks

Having a panic attack can be very painful and scary experience for anyone, although not lethal they do cause overall fear and stress of the next attack only making the Anxiety disorder worse. Many people get so scared of having an attack in public they begin to have one, this is why most people with this condition begin to develop a fear of large crowds.

Panic Attack Symptoms

Racing heart and tingling sensations

Constant chest tightness from anxiety

Dizzy spells resulting to panic

Hot flashes followed up with waves of anxiety

Tightness in chest and throat- shortness of breath

Obsessive worries and unwanted thoughts

Overwhelming fear that the anxiety will push you over the edge?

Feeling disconnected to what is going on around you

If you believe you may suffer from Anxiety disorder or have frequent panic attacks then you need to know this condition can be beaten, many people all over the world have been able to overcome it and so can you.

Chapter 19: Self-Help For Curing Anxiety

Disorders

All people who have got anxiety disorders diagnosed show the similar symptoms. However, most people endure a combination of behavioral, physical and emotional symptoms which often fluctuate and may become worse during the times of pressure. When the symptoms get worse, you may need professional help. But, if you realize that something is not right with your mental well-being, you can try to help yourself in treating the symptoms during the initial stages of any symptoms that are troubling you.

Change Your Perspective to Look at Your Worries

You may think that your anxiety is coming from some outside source-events or people that make you anxious. There might be some circumstances that you face with extreme difficulty. But, the fact is that most of the anxiousness of people takes birth within themselves. The trigger does come from an outer source, but there is an internal dialogue running in your body which upholds the anxiety.

Next time you feel anxious; try to notice that you are communicating with yourself about the events and things you are scared of. You always keep telling yourself that the hazardous events may happen any time. You also try to think about the ways in which you can deal with such situations. In brief, you are trying to find solutions to such problems that are not even in existence. You may think that you are gearing up yourself in advance for the worst scenarios.

Think carefully and deep inside your heart, you also know that your worry and anxiousness is unproductive, which saps your emotional and mental energy without concluding in any problem solving action or strategy. You need to give up the notion that your worry helps you in any way. Then only, you can deal with your mental anxiousness in more creative ways.

It involves confronting irrational straining thoughts, discovering how to suspend worrying, and finding out how you can accept ambiguity of your life.

Get Moving

One of the most effective and natural treatment for anxiety is exercise. It relieves you from stress and tension, boosts mental and physical energy, and helps your brain to release endorphins which are the feel good elements of the brain. You can engage in exercises which make use of all your limbs such as running, walking, dancing and swimming. When you practice any of these exercises, you must focus on the movement of your body and your current feelings of the body, not on your thoughts of anxiety. For instance, when you walk or run, you can focus on your feet thumping the ground, the breathing rhythm or how the wind feels on your skin.

When you add this element of mindfulness to your regime, you are meditating in one form. This helps you to focus on your body and the way it feels while you exercise. It also helps you to recover your health faster and keeps you away from constant worries which keep your mind occupied. There are many people who find rock climbing, weight training, martial arts, and boxing especially effective. These activities require your 100% attention and you have to focus completely on the movements of your body. After all, if you do not focus, you could actually get hurt! And you do not have time for anxiety in such activities. You can start with 10 minute sessions thrice a day, and then increase the duration, say 30 minutes once a day.

Relaxation Techniques

When your body is restless, it is more than a merely a feeling of anxiousness. It is the reaction of your body towards flight or fight to a potential threat. The muscles of your body tense up, your heart starts pounding, your breathing increases, and you feel dizzy. Your body gives completely opposite reactions when you are relaxed. The heart rate calms down, the breathing decreases, deep breaths become easier, the muscles relax and the blood pressure becomes stable. Since it is not possible to feel relaxed and anxious simultaneously, you can use a tactic for relieving from anxiety. You can strengthen the response of relaxation of your body.

Progressive Relaxation of Muscles: This technique includes tensing some groups of muscles in your body systematically and then releasing them. It helps your muscles release tension in the long term. After your body relaxes, the mind will also follow to relax.

Deep Breathing: Anxiety makes you breathe faster. This in turn causes symptoms like breathlessness, dizziness, lightheadedness, tingly feet and hands, etc. Such physical symptoms make you frighten, which further leads to panic and anxiety. However, if you take deep breaths from your diaphragm, you can overturn these signs and calm down.

Meditation: Mindfulness meditation is scientifically proven to modify your brain positively. When you practice meditation regularly, it increases the activity on the left of prefrontal cortex. This area is accountable for the sense of joy and serenity.

Educate Yourself to Quickly Calm Down

People who know that they suffer from generalized anxiety disorder sometimes do not know how they can soothe and calm themselves. However, it is a very easy technique to learn. You can make drastic changes in your life with just one technique. You need to focus on one of your physical senses- hearing, vision, smell, touch or taste. You can also work on more senses if you learn faster. Whenever you observe that the symptoms of your disorder are arising, you can try doing one of the following:

Sight: Look at a beautiful view nearest to you. You can also look at an old family album treasured by you, some art works, watch movies or some funny TV shows, watch light weight documentaries online. Try closing your eyes and visualize a place which is rejuvenating and peaceful. This will boost positive chemicals in your brain and divert your mind from negative thoughts.

Sound: Grab a collection of soothing music and listen to it. Sing along with the tunes of your favorite song. You can also dance to its tunes. Call a school friend. Try to focus on the mesmerizing reverberations of nature- ocean waves hitting the rocks, singing birds, rustling of wind through the trees. You can also procure these sounds online if you do not find them nearby.

Smell: Our nose is a very powerful sensory organ. It can work wonders to calm you down. Light perfumed candles or inhale the scent of flowers in your garden. Go out of your house and breathe fresh and clean air. Spray your favorite perfume without any reason just to make yourself feel good.

Taste: Treat yourself and go to a favorite restaurant or order a delicacy home. Eat the cuisines slowly, savoring every bite.

Take a hot mug of herbal tea or coffee and enjoy it with a brilliant movie.

Touch: Play with your pet, hug your siblings, parents or friends and say thank you to them for being in your life. Their touch on your body and the smile on your face will brighten your life too. Take a soft blanket and wrap yourself in it. Sit for a while in a cool breeze. Enjoy the luxury of a massage on your neck or hands. You can even go to a spa to avail these services. If you cannot afford to pay every time, you can do it yourself. This will not only keep you busy, but also make you feel good.

Movement: Dance with the tunes of your favorite song, go for a run or a walk, jump on your bed and stretch gently. If you have any other physical ailments related to bones or muscles, perform these activities on a milder level.

Bond with Others

It is a crucial part of overcoming any kind of disease, mental or physical ailment. Anxiety disorders worsen only when the patient feels alone or powerless. Connect with people who care about you and go out with them at social places. It calms down your nervous system to diffuse anxiety. Thus, ask for support from people who can meet you frequently, and share your heart without interruption, listens to you but does not judge or criticize you, keeps away from their phone while being with you. It is not difficult to find such people. Look around and you will find them in your spouse, family members, or friends.

The problem with anxiety disorders is that it makes you feel insecure about your relationships.

Determine the Unhealthy Patterns of Relationships: Think about such times how you react when you feel worried about your relationships with different people. Do you tend to test your friends or spouse? Do you withdraw? Do you accuse them? Do you become clingy? When you come to know about your own behavior, you can talk about your feelings to the people you love and discuss about solutions.

Build a Strong System of Support: Human beings are not made to live isolated. Building a strong system of support does not mean that you should have numerous friends. But, you must have some people around you, whom you can count and trust that they will be present when you need them.

Talk When You Need To: Whenever you feel overwhelmed with anxiety, you must talk your heart out with someone who listens to you patiently. This will help you make your tensions appear less threatening.

Avoid People Who are Not Good For You: You must talk to people who make you feel good, not worse. Recognize such people at the earliest. For instance, you might think that your father or mother is the best person to talk to since they are obviously close to you and know you better. But, if by chance, they also happened to suffer from anxiety disorder in the past, they might not be the best people to talk to. You might feel worse talking to some people who do not have a positive approach towards life. Recognize optimistic people and be in constant touch with them. Their optimistic approach will also help you change your perspective towards life.

Chapter 20: Persistence, Discipline And

Potential

To make the results of your efforts stay with you permanently, you have to develop the habit of being proactive. Changing what you've been comfortable with requires a high level of motivation and genuine desire to change. Having the support of a strong social circle will definitely help you.

If motivation and energy is a concern of yours, consider what you might be nutritionally deficient in. You can refer to this book for a list of possible deficiencies that cause lowered energy and motivation, as well as the supplements, natural foods and herbs that boost the neurotransmitters which increase energy and motivation.

Follow the link to: Motivation Boosters: Supercharge Your Brain Chemistry with Natural Foods and Supplements that Increase Motivation

Long-term improvement develops in small increments overtime. Being proactive will keep that process consistent, and will get you to your goals a lot faster. You will also be able to develop and effectively retain a well-rounded set of interests, skills and hobbies. This habit is vital to boosting your character and core confidence.

Chapter 21: Diet And Exercise

You are what you eat, right? Well with anxiety, that is proving to be more and more true. Studies show that certain types of foods not only have a negative effect on the body, but have a negative effect on the helping you manage your anxiety as well.

Diet for Anti-Anxiety

To accompany the supplements of Vitamin B, try and eat foods that are rich in the Vitamin as well. It will work just like the pill that you take, but allow the body to digest is naturally. Red meats, spinach, nuts, legumes, and oranges all have tons of Vitamin B. You know that old saying that turkey makes you sleepy? Well, interestingly enough turkey (and nuts, milk, oats, and soy) are all high in Tryptophan. This chemical is a brain chemical that is turned in to serotonin (a 'feel good' chemical') inside the body.

Unfortunately for all of us coffee drinkers out there, caffeine doesn't help with anxiety. As caffeine is a stimulant, it can help you not only feel more awake, but more anxious as well making it easier for you to become nervous or overwhelmed in stressful situations. It's best to avoid all caffeinated drinks, even sodas, because of the caffeine content.

Sugar doesn't help either. After the initial sugar rush', your body crashes as it produces insulin as it tries to handle the sugar overload. This leaves you feeling cranky, tired, and possibly open to feeling nervous or worried about something.

Alcohol is a big 'no no' if you have anxiety issues. It is a depressant, and as such, can bring on depressive symptoms when consumed. A glass of wine every now and then, but if you are a heavy drinker, there is a good chance that this habit is part of the reason why you are having issues with anxiety.

Run It Off

Exercise has long been used to work off excess stress. And is the number one key factor to assisting with maintaining strong mental grounding as well as physical fitness. It improves alertness, keeps your body in motion so you don't get tired easily, and is a great alternative to worrying.

While 45 minutes of aerobic exercise are great for your physical mental health, sometimes a quick 10-minute walk can get the job done. If you are feeling overwhelmed, anxious, or worrying about something that you can't seem to stop thinking about, go outside and take a walk. Not only will the endorphins your body creates help with the issues, but the rest of the world can act as a distraction and help you sort through your feelings.

Some therapists are even using exercise as a form of therapy, with results saying that one 45-minute exercise session can completely remove symptoms of anxiety for hours afterwards. There is even evidence supporting that a regular workout schedule can lower anxiety levels for some people over a long period of time.

If you don't work out regularly, make a point to try lots of different ideas to get a feel for what you like. Try swimming at your local YMCA or do a Yoga video a couple of times to see how the stretching works for you. Slap on a pair of running shoes and jog or give mountain climbing a shot. Giving yourself multiple options to try until you find something you really like is a great way to make exercise more enjoyable, and if you like what you're doing, you'll be more likely to do it regularly.

Chapter 22: A Brief Look At Meditative

Practices

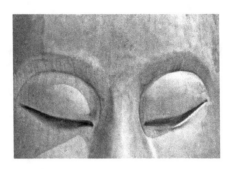

When you begin to do research on meditation, you are going to hear a lot of terms that are specific to the type of meditative practices being considered. For example, chakra is an Indian term that relates to the spiritual center of the human body. Mantra is also associated with Hinduism or Buddhism, although it is not necessary for you to be practicing those religions in order to incorporate this into your meditative practices. As was stated, this report is designed to be free of religious connotations, and although you may have specific religious ideals that you wish to follow, they are not always necessary to enjoy the benefits of meditation. That being said, here are five different types of meditative practices that you may want to consider for your own use.

Focus - One of the guiding principles of many types of meditative practices is to focus your attention by clearing your mind of certain thoughts. In most cases, focus meditation is going to put your mind on a single point of focus—perhaps an object, sound, or thought that allows you to free your mind from the issues that may be stressing you out at the time. Often, this type of meditation may be associated with the use of music, but that is going to be up to you as an individual. It's a good idea for you to experiment with focused meditation to determine how you are going to be able to free your mind of the stressful thoughts that may be plaguing it at the time. Just a few minutes of focused meditation on a daily basis can do wonders for you.

Mindfulness - This is the type of meditation that we are mainly going to focus on in this book. Although you can use the methods that are described in this book to take advantage of any type of meditative practice, you will likely find that mindful meditation is the most beneficial for almost any situation. Rather than emptying your mind of all thoughts, mindful meditation allows you to ponder on the situation that is troubling you or to ponder on something pleasant and peaceful. You can focus on what is around you, such as the sounds or activities that are occurring, allowing your mind to simply flow from one thought to the next. It is not necessary for you to focus on a mantra during this meditative practice. Simply block out the annoyances of the day and allow your mind to flow freely.

Mantra - During this type of meditation, which is often associated with religion, you are going to focus on a word or sound that is chanted during the time that you are meditating. Some people find that this helps them to focus, while others find that it is more of an annoyance. Focusing your mind on that sound or word may help you to let go of some of the stress of your day.

Movement - This type of meditation is often one that is difficult to grasp, but it can have many benefits when you get the hang of it. During movement meditation, you will sit quietly with your mind focused and your eyes closed, concentrating on your breathing patterns. During the time that you are focused on your breathing, you will allow your body to make repetitive movements that flow smoothly, such as moving your arms or swaying from side to side. One of the variations is walking meditation that we will discuss later. Many people find this meditation to be therapeutic, and it is a great way to relax and focus your energies.

Spiritual - I saved this one for last because this book is not about religious meditation. That being said, many people consider a form of spirituality to be separate from religion. During this type of meditation, you use quiet time to focus on your spiritual side and to pray; you allow yourself to be free of other thoughts during this time. You may find this meditation to be relaxing and beneficial in many ways.

The type of meditation that you practice is really up to you. For some people, a combination of practices is best—or they may switch from one form of meditation to another, depending upon their needs. In most cases, it is best for you to master one form of meditation before you decide to move on to another. This way, you will be able to master all of the benefits that are available from each particular meditative practice and enjoy those benefits in your life.

Spiritual vs. Conscientious Meditation

It is noteworthy that although many people meditate for spiritual reasons, it still has benefits that are outside of their spirituality. Meditating regularly can help you to focus your energies and can get you away from the stresses that we all experience on a daily basis. As this world continues to put more and more stress on us, the need to meditate becomes more apparent. By simply spending a few minutes every day on a meditative practice, it can help to calm your nerves and make you more comfortable with the person that you happen to be. It is not always necessary for meditation to be spiritual, and in some cases, it can simply be a matter of focusing your energies to make important decisions. Ultimately, the type of meditation and the focus of the energy is going to be up to you as an individual.

Chapter 23: Understanding The

Symptoms And Causes Of Anxiety

The first part of treating anxiety disorder properly is to understand it. What exactly is anxiety disorder? What causes it? And how would you know if you have it (and thus seek out the appropriate treatment)?

In medical terms, anxiety describes a disorder that causes a patient to feel constantly apprehensive or worried. This kind of mental disorder often affects how an individual behaves and makes decisions, and its sufferers can also reveal physical symptoms. Anxiety disorders range from mild, where the patient constantly feels a prickle of uneasiness, to severe, where the symptoms become so debilitating that they interfere with how the patient is able to handle daily life (e.g., his or her family relationships, school or office work, etc.).

An anxiety disorder may also be present in someone who reacts in a way that is disproportionate to a certain situation. In other words, a patient who frequently ends up becoming far more agitated or disturbed than necessary when they are mildly inconvenienced is usually suffering from anxiety disorder.

However, not all anxiety disorders are the same. Below is a list of the most common anxiety disorders, along with their symptoms:

1.) *Generalized Anxiety Disorder (GAD).* As its name suggests, this variety of anxiety disorder is the most common. An individual with GAD may share the same worries about their finances, family, career or schooling just like everyone else does on occasion. However, the difference is that GAD sufferers often cannot pinpoint what it is exactly they are worried about, and yet they find themselves constantly on edge (to the point that it can be difficult to enjoy the present or even to function normally). Those who suffer from GAD tend to expect failure or tragedy in just about every situation, making them unable to participate in normal school, family, or work activities out of fear that something may go terribly wrong (even when the circumstances don't warrant such).

2.) *Social Anxiety Disorder (SAD)*. This kind of anxiety disorder is characterized by the chronic and often misplaced fear of being embarrassed or judged in a negative light by the public. People who suffer from SAD often get extreme stage fright or a heightened fear of intimacy with those close to them. As a result, they may try to avoid all kinds of social contact to the point where their normal life is severely affected.

3.) *Phobia*. A phobia is characterized by an intense and often irrational fear of a specific situation (e.g., being stuck in a small, enclosed space) or thing (e.g., clowns or spiders). It differs from GAD in the sense that an individual's anxiety attack is triggered by a very specific stimulus, which can cause the patient to try and avoid such at all costs. Although the patient is usually aware that his or her phobia is irrational or absurd, they are still unable to prevent the feeling of anxiety or fear that crops up within them when faced with the object of their phobia.

While some phobias are harmless enough, there are quite a few that can prevent an individual from living a normal life.

4.) *Obsessive Compulsive Disorder*. This variant of anxiety disorder is characterized by repetitive actions or thoughts. OCD sufferers often repeat their actions in a certain pattern, such as washing their hands for a specific number of times or walking down the street so that their feet don't touch the lines on the bricks. Those who suffer from OCD also know that their actions are irrational, but often find themselves becoming increasingly uneasy if they don't carry them out.

5.) *Panic Disorder*. Panic attacks are among the most inconvenient variants of anxiety disorders since they have highly physical and sometimes violent manifestations. A person suffering from a panic attack can suddenly feel an intense burst of terror or nervousness, which is often followed by physical symptoms like dizziness, nausea, as well as breathing difficulties.

As with phobias, panic disorders can be triggered by prolonged exposure to a frightening event or object or even to extreme stress. However, they can also emerge from out of nowhere and can last anywhere between ten minutes to about several hours.

6.) *Post Traumatic Stress Disorder (PTSD)*. PTSD is rooted in a particularly traumatic incident or occurrence in a patient's life, and it is often triggered by exposure to certain kinds of stimuli that may remind the patient of the said event. People who suffer from PTSD often have to endure flashbacks of their painful ordeals, and this may sometimes cause them to behave in a drastically different way towards even their loved ones.

Soldiers who had to fight alongside an army during a brutal war, for example, often end up with PTSD as a result of all the horrors they might have witnessed. Sometime after the Vietnam war, some of the old war veterans suffering from PTSD were noted to scream and to duck for cover whenever they heard an old car sputtering in the street. (The sound made by the car reminded many of the gunshots they heard during the war.)

7.) *Separation Anxiety Disorder*. Often observed in young children attending school for the first time, separation anxiety disorder manifests when a patient becomes excessively disturbed or agitated in instances where s/he is separated from a person or place that makes them feel safe or secure. Young children who have to be separated from their parents for the first time in order to attend class, for example, may exhibit displays of extreme distress such as wailing, throwing tantrums or stubbornly refusing to leave their parent's side.

There are many things that can bring about an anxiety disorder, and sometimes, a combination of them can also result in a patient manifesting symptoms of the said malady:

1.) *Medical Factors*. Anxiety can sometimes go hand in hand with certain medical conditions such as asthma, anemia, or cardiovascular disease, since anxiety episodes can trigger the manifestations of the aforementioned ailments as well as vice versa. The stress that dealing with a serious and life-threatening illness can also saddle a patient with anxiety. Blood clots in the lungs or pulmonary embolisms can also have the same effect since they lead to a lack of oxygen intake, which can make the patient have difficulty breathing (a well-known symptom of an anxiety attack). In certain cases, heightened anxiety can also be attributed to a particularly potent kind of medication as a side effect.

2.) *Heredity and genetics*. Individuals who were born into families with a family history of anxiety or depression have a higher risk of developing anxiety disorder than patients who weren't. Thus, a patient can actually be genetically predisposed to developing and manifesting the symptoms of anxiety disorder.

3.) *Traumatic events*. As with PTSD sufferers, some anxiety disorders are born as a result of experiencing an immensely traumatic event. Being victimized by a violent crime such as rape or attempted murder, losing a loved one, or witnessing and experiencing severe abuse are all instances that could trigger an anxiety disorder.

4.) *Stress*. Everyone experiences stress from time to time, but prolonged and uninterrupted exposure to such is unhealthy. The common factors that anxiety disorder patients often cite as their triggers include stressful difficulties in school, at work, at home, about money, and even in relationships. Drastic changes in one's lifestyle, much like those brought about by events like divorce or separation, can also generate enough stress to make a patient feel anxious.

5.) *Other external factors*. Being in the midst of a devastating natural disaster such as a flood or an earthquake could also bring about an anxiety disorder. Being exposed to high altitudes for too long can also be a trigger for anxiety as the oxygen supply in such a scenario is significantly reduced.

6.) *Substance Abuse*. It has been estimated that about half of the individuals suffering from anxiety are experiencing such as a symptom of either drug or substance addiction or withdrawal. Illegal drugs like amphetamines or cocaine, for instance, have been known to bring about symptoms of anxiety disorders in its users after the initial wave of euphoria has passed. Withdrawing from strong prescription drugs such as barbiturates or benzodiazepines can also incur the same effect upon a patient who is trying to curb their addiction to the said drugs.

7.) *Abnormal brain chemistry*. A healthy human being has normal levels of neurotransmitters in their brain. If your neurotransmitters end up unbalanced, however, then they are unable to function properly. This prevents your brain from reacting as it should in certain scenarios, thus making you more vulnerable to anxiety disorder.

Now that you have a broader understanding of anxiety disorder, its variants, symptoms, and causes, you can move on to reading about ways to deal with it. The most effective way to deal with anxiety usually involves a three-pronged approach, one that involves controlling your diet, lifestyle, and then treating the root of your anxiety. The following chapter will discuss the first item of that approach in detail.

Chapter 24: How To Perform Basic

Tapping

Before we look at various techniques and meridian points for EFT and tapping I highly recommend reviewing the tips below which can be used to enhance all of the techniques and enable you to achieve much better results.

For optimal results from tapping, use all fingertips to tap the meridian points. If you use only two fingers for tapping, you may not be able to cover the meridian points completely.

Make sure you use only your fingertips and not the finger pads for performing tapping. Studies reveal that fingertips have more meridian points compared to finger pads and hence it will help to give you better results.

Make sure you are not wearing any jewelry, watches or glasses as it could significantly hamper the tapping process.

Make sure you apply enough pressure when you are tapping.

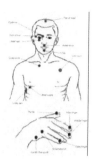

You will need to tap each point for approximately 5 seconds.

How to find the right tapping points to perform EFT and tapping?

You start at the karate chop point along the side of your hand. Either side is fine.

Then you move to the top of your head and work your way down. To be more specific, you could start tapping from the center of the skull to top portion of the back of your head.

Now, tap on your eyebrows by spreading your fingers evenly across the eyebrows.

Once you have tapped on eyebrows, you may continue tapping on the side of your eyes, along the bone next to your eyes.

Now, you may tap beneath your eyes, this area is right above your cheeks.

You may tap on the area beneath your nose.

You also need to tap at your chin point.

Now, you have to tap on the collarbone area as well. (To locate collarbone area, first track down the U-shaped segment seen at the neck bottom and feel the bone in the middle of your chest. Now, move an inch lower from this bone and one inch to both left side and right side.

Tap the area beneath your arm, at about four inches beneath your armpit.

These 9 points form the basis of most of the tapping sessions and after your try it a few times you will be able to remember it easily.

EFT tapping scripts

Now, let us learn about EFT tapping scripts which when coupled with tapping can bring about drastic changes in your life. These are a very important part of the EFT procedure. An affirmative or positive statement is known as EFT tapping script, which helps to get rid of negative energy.

The 5 Step Sequence

This is the core sequence for EFT and tapping:

Analyze the negative feelings or concerns that you wish to solve with the help of EFT. You need to identify all the problems that are affecting you and should be able to identify particular issues.

Once you have identified the issues, you need to rate the problems on scale of 10 (A rating of 10 denotes an issue which you find most difficult to cope with).

Create a setup phrase – A Setup phrase is based on the issue you wish to tackle and includes a positive statement that acknowledges your weakness. For example, "*Even though I have this anxiety, I deeply and completely accept myself*".

Now, you need to tap at your karate chop point and start reciting the setup phrase(s). Then move to the top of the head and work your way down as outlined on the previous page. At each point you say a Reminder Phrase. This is a simplified version of your setup phrase. For example when you tap from the point at the top of your head down to the point under your arm you would say *"This anxiety"* or "This sore knee".

Once you have covered all the meridian points, you need to reassess the intensity of your issue on a scale of 10 to observe and changes.

You can repeat the tapping until you feel that problem is less severe or rates less than two in terms of its intensity.

Also, after you have completed one round, you may modify your setup phrases to bolster you with more confidence. For example, it may be like "I feel better and I will do better".

For a video demonstration with the founder, Gary Craig himself, click here.

How to create your own tapping script?

Obviously, situations and problems vary from person to person and in order to receive the best treatment or create the best practice it's good to have your own personal tapping script. In general it's recommended to follow the pattern:

1) You acknowledge the problem or pain.

2)   You accept yourself in spite of it.

The standard phrase is as follows:

Even though I have this _____, I deeply and completely accept myself.

Example:

Even though I have this fear of needles, I deeply and completely accept myself.

Even though I have this pain in my knee, I deeply and completely love myself.

Of course not all problems or issues will fit nicely into the "Even though I have this _____" sentence. There's no need to worry, EFT allows for a great deal of flexibility. For example you could say *"Even though my knee hurts, I deeply and completely love myself."*

Another important point when creating your own setup script is that it should be aimed at fixing you and your pain, not someone else and what you deem to be there problem. For example, if you have a rather troublesome teenage daughter who causes you nothing but grief your sentence should be more structured around you. The following is an example of a bad setup phrase:

"Even though my daughter is a nightmare, I completely and deeply love myself."

A better setup phrase would be:

"Even though I get frustrated by my daughter, I completely and deeply love myself."

Tips to help improve your positive statements (affirmations)

Below are some techniques that you can use to help you to use your affirmations or positive statements. These are aimed more at improving certain areas of your life rather than fixing problems.

Optimal timing – The best time to perform tapping is when you wake up and before you go to bed. You can also perform tapping at any other time throughout the day but these two times are the most effective.

Do tapping/affirmations in front of the mirror – This helps empower your affirmations and tapping.

Perform tapping on a regular basis and be confident that you will get good result from tapping. By being more optimistic about the results the more likely you are to receive better ones.

Chapter 25: How To Apply Aromatherapy

To Your Everyday Life

When applying the oil formulas, give yourself several minutes of slow, deep, even breathing while you imagine how, with each breath, the oil molecules are entering your bloodstream, and spreading throughout your body, relaxing tight muscles and alleviating tensions and strain. These moments will soon become one of your favorite times of the day.

Regardless of how you use the essential oils, more and more research is showing that aromatherapy does work and it works quickly and effectively to help reduce stress and anxiety. The next time you feel tense and stressed out consider essential oils that relax and sedate including, bergamot, chamomile, lavender, lemon, orange, sandalwood, and Lavender.

Lavender is one of the most popular essential oils and is often referred to as the "universal oil". With its calming, earthy, lightly sweet and freshly floral scent, it is widely beloved for its relaxing and balancing effects on both the physical and emotional bodies. Lavender promotes rest and relaxation, especially when inhaled. It also has antiseptic and anti-inflammatory properties according to Aroma Web, making it a good remedy for acne, eczema and other skin problems.

Some of the other, more popular essential oils used to combat stress and anxiety are:

Chamomile: There are two types of chamomile oil, Roman and German. Roman chamomile is better at treating mental irritation, impatience and PMS while German chamomile is more effective in the treatment of irritated skin. Both types promote overall digestive health and may help calm an upset stomach which can sometimes be a result of anxiety or stress.

Eucalyptus: Eucalyptus oil has a very distinct, strong aroma and can be used to treat a variety of ailments, including headaches. When used in a vaporizer, the oil can help open up sinus passages and relieve coughing, sneezing and other respiratory symptoms. Eucalyptus is a great sleep inducer and will promote a calming atmosphere in order to have a restful slumber.

Peppermint: Peppermint oil, with its candy-like aroma, is a great mind stimulator when inhaled, promoting mental clarity and enhancing focus. It also works wonders on headaches and stomach discomfort. This oil can give a burst of energy, but without the ill effects of caffeine.

Rose: Rose oil is a great multi-purpose oil, but it can be very costly due to the difficult extraction process. It is recommended to use rose oil for treatment of eczema, depression, and stress.

Frankincense: With its comforting warm, exotic aroma, Frankincense's most common use is stress relief; however, it may also be applied topically to the skin to rejuvenate the mind and create a sense of wellbeing.

Vanilla: The pure scent of warm vanilla makes you feel right at home. With the ability to both soothe and promote tranquil relaxation, and stimulate mental clarity.

Index of Herbs and Essential Oils

A. Amber - encourages harmony and balance

Angelica Seed - anchoring, restorative, strengthening, and depression

Aniseed - energizing, toning

B. Balsam Peru - Used on chafed skin to soothe

Basil - deodorant, soothing agent, insect repellent, muscle relaxant

Bay - Amenorrhea, colds, dyspepsia, flu, loss of appetite, tonsillitis

Benzoin - uplifting and soothing

Bergamot - calming, balancing

Birch,Sweet - arthritic and muscular pain and can be a stimulant to circulation

Birch, White - soothing agent, muscle relaxant

C.Cajeput - antiseptic, deodorant, insect repellent

Camphor - balancing, stimulating, toning, cooling

Cardamom - muscle relaxant, skin conditioner, soothing agent

Carrot Seed - muscle relaxant, soothing agent, skin conditioner, aphrodisiac

Cedarwood, Atlas - eases aches and pains

Cedarwood,Texas - aid nervous tension and stress

Chamomile, Blue - soothing, toning

Chamomile, Roman - calming

Cinnamon Leaf - stimulating, energizing

Cistus - stimulating, toning, soothing

Citronella - soothing aroma type

Clary Sage - balancing, calming, toning

Clove Bud - stimulating, energizing

Coriander - warming, stimulating

Cypress- stimulating

D. Dill - reduce appetite

E.Elemi - nervous exhaustion

Eucalyptus - toning, stimulating

Eucalyptus (organic) - deodorant, antiseptic, soothing agent, skin

conditioner, insect repellent
Eucalyptus Citriodora - air freshener and good for clearing
Eucalyptus Radiata - respiratory infections.

Eucalyptus Smithii - painful joints and muscles

F.Fennel Essential - energizing, toning
Fir Needle - aroma of a Christmas tree
Fir Silver Needle - refresh the aroma of a Christmas tree

Frankincense - stimulating, toning, grounding

G. Galbanum - skin conditioner, muscle relaxant

Geranium - balancing, soothing skin type: oily, dry

Geranium (organic) - skin refresher, astringent

Ginger - energizing, warming
Grapefruit - energizing

H. Helichrysum - clear the mind, chest and sinus and relieves aches, pains and menstrual discomfort

Ho Essential Oil - balancing, stimulating,

toning, cooling

Hyssop - warming, stimulating, balancing

J.Jasmine - uplifting, balancing

Juniper Berry (organic) - energizing

K. Kanuka - For the relief of swelling and muscular pain, for sprains, strains and sports injuries

L. Lavandin - soothing agent, muscle relaxant, skin conditioner, astringent

Lavandin (organic) - stimulating, energizing

Lavender 40/42 - calming, balancing, soothing

Lavender, E. Europe - calming, balancing, soothing

Lavender, High Alpine - muscle relaxant, soothing agent , balancing, soothing

Lemon - energizing, uplifting, antiseptic, soothing agent

Lemongrass - calming

Lime - energizing, uplifting

Linden Blossom Absolute - calming and stress reduction and a tonic for the nervous system

M. Mandarin, Red - calming

Mandarin, Red (organic) - soothing agent, astringent, skin conditioner

Manuka - muscular pain relief

Marjoram - calming

Marjoram, (organic) - calming

Melissa - uplifting effect on mind and body

Myrrh - toning, stimulating, soothing

N. Neroli - antiseptic, emollient

Niaouli - body aches and pains

Nutmeg - energizing, stimulating, warming

O Oak Moss Absolute - calming

Orange - astringent, soothing agent, skin conditioner

Orange, (organic) - calming

Oregano - relieves muscle aches and pains and assists in increasing energy

P. Palmarosa - insect repellent, skin conditioner, soothing agent, emollient, muscle relaxant

Patchouli - anti-inflammatory agent, antiseptic, astringent, aphrodisiac, perfume

Pepper, Black - muscle relaxant, aphrodisiac

Peppermint - energizing, stimulating

Peppermint (organic) - insect repellent, emollient, antiseptic, muscle relaxant

Petitgrain - calming

Pine Needle (Scotch Pine) - It has a deodorant affect and is often used in commercial preparations

R.Ravensara - loosening tight muscles, relieving menstrual discomfort and aches and pains

Rose Absolute - cooling, balancing, calming, toning

Rose Geranium - balancing, soothing skin type: oily, dry

Rose Otto - cooling, balancing, calming, toning

Rosemary - antiseptic, muscle relaxant, soothing agent, skin conditioner

Rosewood - Relaxing and deodorizing

S. Sage - soothing agent

Sandalwood - calming, grounding

Scotch Pine (Pine Needle) - Stimulates, refreshes and cleanses

Spearmint - calming

Spearmint (organic) - insect repellent, emollient, astringent, soothing agent, muscle relaxant

Spruce - Coughing, depression

T.Tagetes - Corns, warts

Tangerine - astringent for oily skin

Tea Tree - energizing, stimulating, toning

Tea Tree (organic) - insect repellent, antiseptic

Thyme, Linalol - energizing, stimulating, toning

Thyme, White - energizing, stimulating, toning

V.Vanilla Absolute - emollient, aphrodisiac

Vetiver - emollient

Y. Yarrow - chest infections, digestive problems and nervous exhaustion

Ylang Ylang - calming, balancing

Chapter 26: Learning To Follow Through

The great thing about small talk is that no matter how fleeting or spontaneous they are, they remain meaningful when you want them to. What usually start out as a light and casual conversation can actually blossom into something great. And that's where your skill in following through comes in.

Some small talks are better left as that: conversations with random people that you'll never meet again. But then there are also those that prompt you to seek a follow through. When you feel an immediate connection or a spark with the person you're talking with, you do not want to let that moment stay as a fleeting memory from the past. You want to take a proactive approach in building a connection with that person.

During the course of your conversation, pay particular attention to what is being said and see if there's anything you want to build up on. For example, if you are a business owner and you found out that the person you are having small talk with can actually introduce you to people in the industry, then you'd want to establish a connection with this person. This is called networking, which is critical in business.

Shared interests

Sometimes shared interests can be a good reason, too, for keeping in touch. If both of you share a mutual passion for books, for example, you may want to exchange notes on a few books or organizations for readers. Most people have social networking accounts anyway, so you can take your discussion further online and possibly meet up again in the future.

If you are out looking for a date, one way of doing it is by initiating small talk with the person of your interest. Remember the strategies outlined in the previous chapters and you should be fine. The key is to make it casual, not awkward or weird. You want to establish an immediate connection, present yourself as someone likable, and pique the interest of your romantic prospect to make him or her want to see you again.

But most importantly, always be sensitive about the timing or appropriateness of initiating small talk. These kind of things are best enjoyed when there is a mutual agreement that you are both open to talking as signified by body language and overall demeanor. Don't push if it isn't meant to be.

In sum, small talks may seem inconsequential, but when done right and with the right attitude, they can become an excellent bridge connecting us to people whom we wouldn't have otherwise met had we chosen not to bother. They are also the perfect exercise in overcoming our fears and anxieties, particularly in social situations.

So the next time you find yourself in a position to initiate small talk, do so. You'll never where it can take you.

Chapter 27: Symptoms Of And Causes Of

Anxiety Disorders

Anxiety attacks are characterized by episodes of fear without a warning and reach a peak where you feel total lack of control or about to die. Due to the physical impact of many anxiety disorders, you may confuse anxiety with other conditions such as cardiac arrest. Let's take a look at the most common anxiety indicators that should make you seek immediate help:

*Uncontrollable feelings of panic, fear and obsessive thoughts

*Choking sensation, breathing problems and heart palpitations

*Sudden feeling of losing control or about to die

*Persistent nightmares, chills and hot flashes

*Intrusive or painful memories

*Overwhelming panic, shaking or trembling

*Stomach cramps, nausea and muscle tension

I am sure that you would want to know the causes of various anxiety disorders in order to solve the problem from the core so let us have a look at some common causes of anxiety disorders. You will realize that most of these causes are similar to the causes of depression.

What Causes Anxiety Disorders?

For now, the actual cause of anxiety disorders is not known, only for the triggers such as traumatic events. However, anxiety disorders may run in families where environmental factors may act on your genes to trigger an attack. Brain chemistry may also play a part in causing panic attacks. The following are risk factors associated with anxiety:

Trauma

If you have faced trauma or past abuse, you are at a higher risk of developing anxiety disorders. Traumatic factors affect both children and adults.

Personality

You could be having certain personality types, which tend to be more prone to anxiety disorder. Such traits could be resulting from brain chemistry. For instance, if you are a people pleaser, a perfectionist, are highly sensitive and highly performance conscious, you are likely to have an anxiety disorder.

Genetics

Your close family members or parents could be having an anxiety disorder gene that can be transferred to you.

Related health disorders

Mental problems such as depression can often cause you to experience an anxiety disorder as well.

Stress

Major stressors such as looking for a job, a death in the family, difficulty in relationships or debts can lead to excessive anxiety. Stress may also result from chronic illnesses that can cause anxiety over your future life or treatment costs.

Chapter 28: Nutritional Methods Of

Dealing With Anxiety

Foods (and Drinks) To Enjoy
Eat Whole Foods – Whole foods are foods that are unrefined and unprocessed or very little of either. Some examples are vegetables, fruits, non-homogenized dairy

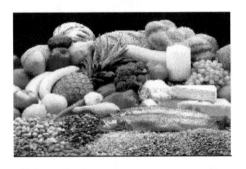

products, so-called unpolished grains, etc. Aside from helping reduce (or even prevent some) anxiety, these foods help your body create protective substances for itself.

Eat Legumes – Legumes are things such as soy beans, peas, lentils, etc. These contain an essential called amino acid called lysine.

Eat Grains – Containing another essential amino acid known as methionine, grains coupled with legumes are a well-rounded solution, especially for vegetarians.

Eat Red Meat – A good way to remember what red meats are, is to obviously note that the color of the meat is red in its raw state. Furthermore, red meat darkens when it's cooked. It's a good source of protein and amino acids. Some examples are beef, rib roast, rabbit, lamb and veal.

Eat Poultry & Eggs – Chicken, turkey, duck, dove and quail are some examples. Poultry and eggs provide another good source of protein and contain lost of needed vitamins and minerals.

Eat Fish – Yet another source of protein, fish contains fewer calories than meat and contains omega-3 fatty acids which are good for your heart.

Eat & Drink Dairy Products – Milk, cheese, yogurt and other dairy products are an excellent source of calcium. They lower the risks of some types of cancer.

Foods (and Drinks) To Avoid

Empty Calorie Foods – Empty Calorie Foods are foods that have little or no nutritional value. Some examples are French fries, chips, ice cream, soda and sweetened fruit drinks.

Caffeine – Caffeine is a stimulant. Anxiety is the sudden rush of adrenaline creating a fight-or-flight response. A stimulant is the last thing you want. Put that chocolate, energy drink, certain teas and coffee down!

Alcohol – Alcohol adversely affects brain function, mood, perception and behavior. When dealing with anxiety, drinking alcohol is the last thing you want.

Avoid Nicotine. It starts out as a stimulant and it develops into a depressant. Back away from the tobacco, in all forms.

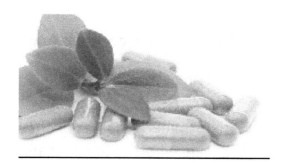

Chapter 29: Ways To Reduce Stress And

Anxiety

Once you determine your personal stressors and decide whether to eliminate, minimize, or cope with each stressor, you are ready to move on to the next stress management step. Psychologists have some practical suggestions for minimizing stress in your life. By incorporating a healthy mindset, cultivating certain habits, and incorporating stress-reducing activities into your daily routine, you will greatly lower the negative stress in your life.

Stress-Reducing Habits and Activities

Learn to say "no"
Do not overcommit yourself. It is ok to say no to certain activities that are good but not necessary to your personal goals.

Do something fun every day
Schedule time each day to do something you enjoy, even if it is just for 20-30 minutes. Whether that is crafting, playing

a sport, practicing an instrument, or reading a book, doing something that you like each day will help counteract any negative stress you experienced that day.

Schedule in relaxation time
Try to leave open time slots in your schedule to allow for sufficient relaxation and down time.

Schedule in vacation time
Try to schedule in regular days off of work, in between holidays. Taking a longer vacation like 5-7 days in the spring or summer is another great way to relieve stress and avoid work burnout.

Prioritize Sleep
Make sure that you get at least 8 hrs of sleep each night. This will keep your body and mind healthy and will help you to have a balanced perspective during the day.

Exercise regularly
Try to exercise for 20 minutes each day or more. Raising your heart rate will not only burn calories but will boost your endorphins and help burn off stress.

Eat   healthy   foods
Avoid junk foods, carbs, and foods that are high in fat. Fruits, veggies, and whole grains are great options for helping you to feel your best.

Express   your   feelings
Talking to a friend or therapist, or writing in a journal are great ways to help express yourself. Self-expression is necessary for releasing the emotions and stress that have accumulated during the day.

Connect   with   other   people
Schedule time to socialize and visit with friends on a regular basis. Expressing yourself and learning to see things from another point of view are effective at lowering stress.

Change   your   perspective
Commit to thinking positively. Pick out the good in every situation. Try to see every opportunity as a chance for growth.

Have   reasonable   expectations
Avoid stressing yourself out by having unrealistic standards or expectations. Instead, try to set realistic and moderate

goals for projects, for yourself, and for a given situation.

Try yoga
Yoga not only helps increase your strength and flexibility, but controlled breathing exercises can help lower your heart rate and reduce stress.

Schedule solitude
Many individuals help lower their stress by incorporating meditation, prayer, and moments of silence into their daily routine.

Conclusion

Thank you again for downloading this book!

I hope this book was able to help you learn more about social anxiety and find ways on how to overcome it so you can open yourself up to greater possibilities.

The next step is to apply what you have learned in this book. Until you fully apply what you have learned, the information has not power! World renowned speaker and best-selling author, Tony Robbins often says 'Knowledge is not enough. You must take action!' It is not through acquiring new information that the quality of our lives improve, but through taking new actions, so I encourage you from the bottom of my heart to take action on what you have learned here and believe me, the only problem you'll have is that you didn't read this book 6 months ago and take action then!

Finally, if you enjoyed this book, please take the time to share your thoughts and post a review on Amazon. It'd be greatly appreciated!

Thank you and good luck!

Printed in the USA
CPSIA information can be obtained
at www.ICGtesting.com
LVHW010857160324
774655LV00033B/1129